Contents

Part 1: Breast Development   1

Questions 1–8 discuss common questions about breast development, such as:
- What are breast buds?
- What are signs of breast problems in my daughter?
- What are some tips for buying my daughter's first bra?

Part 2: Menstruation   9

Questions 9–20 review the menstrual cycle, including facts about common symptoms and other related body changes girls experience when their menstrual cycle begins:
- When should I expect my daughter to have her first period?
- What symptoms will my daughter experience during her periods?
- What menstrual issues should prompt me to take my daughter to a doctor?

Part 3: Sanitary Pads and Tampons   21

Questions 21–31 explain the differences between sanitary pads and tampons, as well as when they are appropriate to use:
- What should my daughter know about sanitary pads?
- When should my daughter use tampons?
- What is my daughter's risk of getting TSS and how can she avoid it?

Part 4: Hygiene   35

Questions 32–37 discuss the importance of hygiene as your daughter continues to grow during puberty:
- Should my adolescent daughter use antiperspirants or deodorants?
- Why is my daughter starting to suffer from acne?
- As a mother of a daughter entering puberty, what skin care advice can I give her?

100 Questions & Answers About Your Daughter's Sexual Wellness and Development

Carolyn F. Davis, MD, FACOG

Assistant Professor
Department of Obstetrics and Gynecology
Virginia Commonwealth University
School of Medicine
Inova Campus
Falls Church, VA

JONES AND BARTLETT PUBLISHERS
Sudbury, Massachusetts
BOSTON   TORONTO   LONDON   SINGAPORE

2050 58200

World Headquarters

Jones and Bartlett Publishers
40 Tall Pine Drive
Sudbury, MA 01776
978-443-5000
info@jbpub.com
www.jbpub.com

Jones and Bartlett Publishers
Canada
6339 Ormindale Way
Mississauga, Ontario L5V 1J2
Canada

Jones and Bartlett Publishers
International
Barb House, Barb Mews
London W6 7PA
United Kingdom

Jones and Bartlett's books and products are available through most bookstores and online
booksellers. To contact Jones and Bartlett Publishers directly, call 800-832-0034,
fax 978-443-8000, or visit our website, www.jbpub.com.

Substantial discounts on bulk quantities of Jones and Bartlett's publications are available to
corporations, professional associations, and other qualified organizations. For details and
specific discount information, contact the special sales department at Jones and Bartlett via
the above contact information or send an email to specialsales@jbpub.com.

The author, editor, and publisher have made every effort to provide accurate information.
However, they are not responsible for errors, omissions, or for any outcomes related to the use
of the contents of this book and take no responsibility for the use of the products and procedures described. Treatments and side effects described in this book may not be applicable to all
people; likewise, some people may require a dose or experience a side effect that is not described
herein. Drugs and medical devices are discussed that may have limited availability controlled by
the Food and Drug Administration (FDA) for use only in a research study or clinical trial.
Research, clinical practice, and government regulations often change the accepted standard in
this field. When consideration is being given to use of any drug in the clinical setting, the health
care provider or reader is responsible for determining FDA status of the drug, reading the package insert, and reviewing prescribing information for the most up-to-date recommendations on
dose, precautions, and contraindications, and determining the appropriate usage for the product. This is especially important in the case of drugs that are new or seldom used.

Production Credits

Executive Publisher: Christopher Davis
Editorial Assistant: Sara Cameron
Associate Production Editor: Leah Corrigan
Associate Marketing Manager: Marion Kerr
Manufacturing and Inventory Supervisor:
  Amy Bacus

Cover Designer: Carolyn Downer
Cover images: © Rubberball Productions;
  © Konstantin Sutyagin/ShutterStock, Inc.;
  © Monkey Business Images/
  ShutterStock, Inc.
Composition: Glyph International
Printing and Binding: Malloy, Inc.
Cover Printing: Malloy, Inc.

Library of Congress Cataloging-in-Publication Data
Davis, Carolyn F.
  100 questions and answers about your daughter's sexual wellness and development / Carolyn
F. Davis.
    p. cm.
  Includes index.
  ISBN 978-0-7637-8545-1 (alk. paper)
  1. Teenage girls—Health and hygiene. 2. Puberty. 3. Adolescence. I. Title. II. Title: One
hundred questions and answers about your daughter's sexual wellness and development.
  RA777.25.D38 2011
  613.9—dc22   2010006912

6048

Printed in the United States of America
14 13 12 11 10   10 9 8 7 6 5 4 3 2 1

Contents

v

I've been a gynecologist and obstetrician for almost two decades. Throughout my years in medicine, whether it's been during my time in medical school, residency, or private practice, I've always been fascinated by the topic of the health, sexual development, and emotional well-being of adolescent girls.

In fact, for nearly 20 years I've extensively researched this topic, attended numerous presentations, written and lectured about it, conferred with a multitude of my medical colleagues, and served as the physician for so many teenaged girls that I've lost count. However, only recently did I undergo a life-changing event that brought all of the dry information, the impersonal clinical data, and the cold, antiseptic facts into a whole new perspective.

My own daughter entered her adolescent years.

As a mother of an adolescent daughter yourself, you know exactly how I feel. The "experts" are good at talking about complex theories, academic statistics, and broad generalities. But when you're personally confronted with the many challenges that arise during your own daughter's adolescence, what you want more than anything else is practical advice and solid information. And that's why I've written this book.

In these pages, I provide you with a lot of medical information. But what's more, I've distilled for you the knowledge, insights, and tips I've learned over the many years that I've concentrated on issues facing adolescent girls. I cover not only issues such as birth control and sexually transmitted diseases but also topics such as how to pick out a girl's first bra, how a girl can learn to easily insert a tampon, and what every girl needs to know about body piercings and tattoos.

In this book I also talk about how you can help your daughter make the right choices during her teen years. My goal is to make your daughter's adolescent years a little less perplexing. And in the end, I hope that means they'll be a whole lot more fun—for both of you.

When my daughter turned eight, I first began to see brief flashes of the woman she was likely to become. Although I absolutely cherished her sweet innocence at that age, I also knew that when she asserted her independence, that was the right course for her to take. After all, butterflies are meant to take flight.

But at the same time, my protective side as a mother was always just beneath—and often, fully above—the surface. Girls today face tremendous pressures. Our society often imposes stressful and unrealistic expectations on them. As a consequence, they can lose their self confidence, and they can also lose their way.

That's when we moms need to make sure that we are an integral part of our daughters' lives. It's a pretty daunting world out there for girls and young women, one that constantly barrages them with thoughts, words, and images of sex, sex, and more sex, but then completely ignores the critical facts about sexual development, sexual health, and sexual protection. Therefore, as mothers, we need to make sure that our daughters have the proper tools and knowledge so that they can become safe, self-confident, and self-fulfilled young women in these difficult times. And we can only do so if we, ourselves, know the facts.

So just remember, even when your young daughter looks all grown up on the outside, on the inside she's still just a vulnerable girl who is facing an often hostile world and who needs your wisdom and guidance. And also remember that even when your teenaged daughter seems to keep pushing you away, she still needs—and wants—your advice and support.

I realize that providing information and assistance to your daughter won't always be easy for you. However, as I always say when I give talks on this subject, being a mom to an adolescent girl reminds me of the slogan they use for the Peace Corps: "It's the toughest job you'll ever love."

PART ONE

Breast Development

What are breast buds?

What are signs of breast problems in my daughter?

What are some tips for buying my daughter's first bra?

More . . .

As we all know, breast development is the most visible sign that a girl is beginning her journey into womanhood. As a result, it has added significance in every girl's life. Along with her hair and skin, your daughter is more likely to focus on her breasts than on any other part of her body. (The boys in your daughter's class are certain to share her fascination with this subject.)

As a mom, you have two goals when it comes to your daughter's breast development. The first is to ensure that she has no breast-related health problems. Luckily, as I'll explain below, you really don't have too much to worry about on that score. But your second goal is much more difficult. Namely, you need to do everything you can to ensure that your daughter has a positive self-image of her body, regardless of whether her breasts are large or small, narrow or full, late in developing or early to show.

It's no secret that our society seems fixated on breasts. As women, we can't ignore the fact that they represent an obvious sign not only of our sex but also of our sexuality. But we can't let breast size and breast development define who our daughters are or how they feel about themselves.

As a physician, the first question I'm always asked about breast development is, "What's normal?" Well, the answer is, "There's a *lot* of variation." However, there are certain facts that are helpful for you to know so that you can keep your daughter informed. Additionally, these facts will help you recognize those rare and unlikely situations where you may need to consult with your daughter's pediatrician about this issue.

1. What are breast buds?

In the medical community, the breast development process is referred to as "**thelarche**," which is pronounced

---

In the medical community, the breast development process is referred to as "thelarche," which is pronounced "thee-LAR-key."

Thelarche

The development of breast tissue in an adolescent.

"thee-LAR-key." (This term can come in handy if you ever want to research the issue on the Internet. If you type in "thelarche," you'll be directed to good, informative medical Web sites. However, if you type in any search term that includes the words "women's breasts," you'll be directed to Web sites that will make you blush.)

The word "thelarche" is a Greek word that simply means "beginning of breast development." This process starts with breast budding, which usually happens when a girl is between the ages of 8 and 10. However, some girls' **breast buds** appear significantly later in **puberty**, and as surprising as it may seem, breast development that begins as early as age 3 may not be deemed abnormal.

The appearance of breast buds will typically occur around the same time that your daughter undergoes a **growth spurt**. This budding process begins when a hormone known as **estradiol** starts coursing through your daughter's body. It's this hormone that causes your daughter's once boy-like figure to begin hinting at its future femininity.

2. What should I do if one of my daughter's breasts is bigger than the other?

Breast buds are tender, raised bumps that appear directly under a girl's nipples. It's not unusual for breast buds to appear on just one side first. As a result, there have been many frantic but unnecessary trips to the doctor when a lump has suddenly appeared under a single nipple of a young girl.

Similarly, a mother can understandably become concerned when one side of her daughter's chest is noticeably larger than the other. (For reasons that are

Breast buds

The early breast tissue that first appears in adolescence.

Puberty

The period of time in which a child undergoes physiological and emotional changes that help her/him develop into a young adult capable of reproducing.

Growth spurt

A period of rapid growth in height, weight, and muscle mass that takes place in adolescence, typically between the ages of 11–14 for girls, and 12–16 for boys.

Estradiol

An estrogen hormone produced by the ovaries that is responsible for breast development and menstrual cycles in females.

Approximately 25% of adolescent girls experience breast asymmetry that persists into adulthood.

not entirely understood, this usually occurs on a girl's left side.) This is not uncommon. Approximately 25% of adolescent girls experience breast asymmetry that persists into adulthood. Later in life, corrective measures can be taken to "even out" this difference in the size of a woman's breasts. (However, the difference between each breast is typically not that noticeable.)

3. What can my daughter do to relieve breast pain?

Unfortunately, breast pain or discomfort is common in adolescent girls. It usually happens in cycles and occurs just before she menstruates. Research has shown that this pain can be increased if a girl drinks anything with caffeine in it, whether it's coffee, soda, or an energy drink. (And, as a further incentive not to use cigarettes, you should let your daughter know that smoking also tends to increase breast pain.)

A breast surgeon I know tells his patients who experience breast pain to avoid caffeinated products, chocolate, and peanuts; to use over-the-counter medications such as **acetaminophen** and **ibuprofen** as needed; and to wear only well-fitted, supportive bras. That's good advice for all of us women. (Except for the "no chocolate" part, of course.)

4. What are signs of breast problems in my daughter?

Once your daughter develops breast buds, she may experience nipple discharge. This is usually caused by irritation to the area, or by an elevated level of the hormone **prolactin**. Increased hormone levels may be the result of medications your daughter is taking or by a growth on her **pituitary gland**. Therefore, if your

Acetaminophen

A common over-the-counter medication used to decrease pain and reduce fevers. This medication is helpful for headaches and menstrual cramps. A common brand name is Tylenol.

Ibuprofen

A commonly used over-the-counter antiprostaglandin medication that helps menstrual cramps. Two common brand names are Motrin and Advil.

Prolactin

A hormone secreted by the pituitary gland that stimulates breast milk production.

Pituitary gland

A gland in the brain that is responsible for producing various hormones.

daughter experiences nipple discharge, you should take her to your pediatrician to be evaluated.

Your daughter may also develop a mass in her breast, even at a young age. Thankfully, the vast majority of these growths are completely benign. Although a trip to the doctor's office is necessary to evaluate the mass, biopsies of the area are greatly frowned-upon by doctors because of the risk of damaging a girl's breast bud. In almost all instances, the masses resolve themselves, remain without causing any problems, or disappear with the use of antibiotics.

One thing you can feel good about is the fact that breast **cancer** is extremely rare in adolescents. In fact, studies show that from 1998 to 2002, the incidence of breast cancer in females below the age of 20 was 0 cases for every 100,000 people. That's right; zero cases. Now, that doesn't mean it never happens, but it's not something that you should spend your time worrying about.

5. When should my daughter start wearing a training bra?

Your young daughter may initially be oblivious to her own breast bud development. For instance, she may put on a clingy shirt and yet have no idea that it's accentuating the breast buds that have seemingly sprung up overnight. That's a good time for you to gently suggest it's time for her to wear a training bra.

At first your daughter may resist the idea. However, eventually she'll grow accustomed to the notion that she ought to wear a bra on certain occasions, such as when she has phys-ed at school. She'll realize that the extra support makes her more comfortable during running and strenuous activities. (She'll also learn that

Cancer
An abnormal growth of cells that impairs normal body function. Also known as malignant tumors, these growths can occur in almost any organ system.

In fact, studies show that from 1998 to 2002, the incidence of breast cancer in females below the age of 20 was 0 cases for every 100,000 people.

sweaty shirts can make breast buds look as if they magically grew.) Before long you'll be off shopping together, looking for a new bra.

Donna says:

I have a daughter who is 11 years old who started wearing white camisoles under her shirts/blouses at age 6. Once I realized that she started to develop breast buds at the age of 9, and they were noticeable under her shirts, she and I sat down and discussed this phase of her adolescent development. I explained to her that when she wears certain shirts, you can tell she is developing breasts and it was time for her to start wearing a training bra. She and I spent a day together and went shopping for her first training bra. There were a lot of choices and it can be overwhelming for a young girl. I measured my daughter's chest before we went out to purchase a training bra. This helped to give us an idea on what size training bra to start with and made her feel more comfortable with the process.

6. What are some tips for buying my daughter's first bra?

If you're about to embark on your first experience buying a bra for your daughter, there are certain things you should know to make the task easier. First, the term "training bra" doesn't have a precise definition. It just generally refers to any bra that is designed for a girl with little if any breast tissue. Some training bras are merely camisoles with an extra panel, some are like sports bras and are simple pieces of stretchy fabric, and others have a small cup with them.

Second, as you know, women's bras have two numbers or sizes: a band size and a cup size. However, most training bras have only one size, starting at 28 and going to 36, and do not have a cup size. In order to determine the size of the bra your daughter needs, first measure in inches the circumference around your daughter's chest just under her breasts. Then, if this is an even number, add 4 inches. If it's an odd number, add 5 inches. This is the correct training bra size to look for.

If your daughter has developed enough breast tissue so that she needs a bra with a cup, you will need to make an additional measurement. You can determine her cup size by measuring her around her chest at the fullest point of her breasts. You then subtract the band number from this larger number. You will end up with a number that is anywhere between one-half an inch to 10 inches (and, on rare occasions, more than 10 inches). At the store or on the Internet, you'll be able to find a chart that converts the number you've calculated to a specific cup size. For instance, "AA" refers to the smallest cup size.

Needless to say, it will be far more convenient if you take the time to determine your daughter's bra size before leaving home. Trying to guesstimate your daughter's bra size in a crowded store while she's cringing with embarrassment and trying to disappear into the floor isn't likely to be too productive. (This will be particularly true if your son proceeds to provide a running commentary of the event for all his fellow shoppers.)

Unfortunately, however, it's been my experience after browsing in many different stores that there is very little consistency among manufacturers when it comes to bra size. Therefore, despite your best efforts, you still may need to have your daughter try on a bunch of them to get the perfect fit. In doing so, it would be very helpful to find a store that caters to girls and has helpful sales associates. (It also would be helpful to leave your son at home.)

7. How large will my daughter's breasts get?

Once a girl's breasts begin developing, she understandably will be interested in how big they'll become. However, there's no surefire way to predict. What you can explain to your daughter is that breast size is mainly determined by genetics. As a consequence, there is no potion she can drink and no lotion she can apply that will noticeably affect the size of her breasts. (Trust me, if anyone develops such a product, it will be all over the news!)

8. Should my adolescent daughter consider breast implants?

If your daughter raises the issue of breast implants, please talk to her candidly and fully about it. Let her know your own thoughts and values regarding this issue. Make sure she realizes that all the Hollywood images of buxom babes don't reflect reality.

And importantly, while being understanding and supportive, make it clear to your daughter that as long as she is an adolescent, you will not even consider letting her get breast implants. Explain to your daughter that getting breast implants involves expensive, invasive surgery. Therefore, it's not something to be taken lightly. Moreover, you should point out that most plastic surgeons will not even consider performing breast surgery on someone who is not an adult. And finally, you should talk to your daughter about feeling positive about the development of her breasts, no matter what their size.

PART TWO

Menstruation

When should I expect my daughter to have
her first period?

What symptoms will my daughter experience
during her periods?

What menstrual issues should prompt me to
take my daughter to a doctor?

More . . .

As I noted earlier, the beginning of breast development is a tremendously important milestone in every girl's life. However, it pales in comparison to the onset of **menstruation**.

Menstruation
The breakdown and shedding of the uterine lining resulting in the menstrual period.

Menstruation. Just hearing the word uttered publicly seems to cause some fully-grown women to squirm with discomfort. And yet, it's a fact of life for all of us. As a result, we have the responsibility of making it crystal clear to our daughters that there is absolutely no need to be ashamed or embarrassed about it.

At the same time, however, we have to be realistic. No matter how much information we provide to our daughters, and no matter how supportive we may be, the onset of menstruation (doctors refer to it as "**menarche**," which is pronounced "MEN-ar-kee") is very likely to be a significant source of concern for any girl.

Menarche
The initial onset of menstrual cycles.

(Just pause and reflect for a moment. When your daughter learns about menstruation, or when she experiences it herself for the first time, she likely will be thinking, "Wait a minute. I'm going to be *bleeding*? From *there*? *Frequently*? For *decades* to come? And it probably will be accompanied by *pain, cramps, and bloating*? *You have got to be KIDDING me!*")

As always, it's crucial for us as mothers to carefully guide our daughters through this unsettling change in life. The best way to do so is by serving as good role models. How we react when the subject of menstruation is raised, and how we react to the onset of our own periods, is likely to be mimicked by our daughters.

Menstruation is truly a strange topic. Even though it's commonplace, it's a taboo subject in the mass media.

Further, whether you realize it or not, even well-educated and well-informed men are completely clueless when it comes to the facts of menstruation. To them, periods are some great female mystery. We need to ensure that our daughters don't perpetuate this misconception that menstruation somehow makes us alien beings.

Clearly, we already have made great advances in that regard. In some cultures in the past, menstruating women were viewed as "unclean" and were segregated from the larger group. We've come a long way since then. But even today, when women are assertive in making their views known or in protecting their own interests, they too often are characterized as suffering from "**PMS**." We have to work in common cause with our daughters to remove this unfair and unfortunate stigma.

9. What do I need to know about my daughter's first menstrual cycle?

Typically, a girl's first **menstrual cycle** is preceded by pubic hair growth. This should serve as a sign to you that your daughter's menstruation is not too far away. Pubic hair growth typically occurs when a girl is about 10 years old. Growth of underarm hair usually follows about 2 years later. Girls have their largest growth spurt during this time period, and menstruation typically begins as well.

All of these developments are the result of new **hormones** swirling around in a girl's body. These hormones are also a primary cause of the emotional roller coaster that girls experience at this age. You may very well notice an increase in your daughter's irritability, moodiness, and even anxiety. Such reactions can first be seen at age 7 with an initial small rise of hormones,

Menstruation

PMS

An abbreviation that refers to premenstrual syndrome. PMS refers to the period of time preceding the menstrual period where, due to elevated levels of progesterone, symptoms of bloating, moodiness, irritability, acne, and breast tenderness are more prevalent.

Menstrual cycle

The monthly episode of vaginal bleeding that can last for up to a week.

Pubic hair growth typically occurs when a girl is about 10 years old.

Hormones

Chemicals produced by an organ that have an effect on other organs or cells in the human body.

Estrogen

Refers to a number of "female" hormones found in the human body. They are produced by the ovaries, but synthetic forms also can be manufactured for use in birth control pills and for other medical purposes.

Adrenal glands

The glands in the human body responsible for producing stress response hormones, such as cortisol and adrenaline. Some androgens, or male-like hormones, are produced in the adrenal glands as well. The adrenal glands lie next to the kidneys.

Androgens

Hormones that cause masculinizing effects such as acne, increased hair growth on the face or body, enlargement of the clitoris, and deepening of the voice. In females, androgens are produced by the adrenal glands and the ovaries.

Growth hormones

Chemicals produced by the pituitary gland that influence metabolism and cause growth of organs.

and then they spike around age 11 when the hormones go into high gear. (When that happens, your previously well-adjusted, good-natured, sweet young daughter may be a little less pleasant to be around.)

These hormones are part of an intricate biological dance within your daughter's body. First, hormones begin to rise from a girl's pituitary gland. These hormones then cause increased **estrogen** to be produced by the girl's ovaries. Next the **adrenal glands** kick in, producing **androgens**. (Androgens are male-like hormones that contribute to hair growth in the pubic region and under the arms.) And finally, **growth hormones** go into their most active stage.

Interestingly, girls typically have their greatest growth spurt about two years before boys do. If you visit any fifth or sixth grade classroom, you're almost certain to notice that the girls are, on average, taller than the boys.

Donna says:

My daughter started her menstrual cycle this year at 11 years old. On the day that she started, we were out visiting a zoo and she complained that she had cramps from all the walking and wasn't feeling well. Later that evening, she called me into the bathroom and indicated that she thought she had started her period. I informed her that she did. She and I sat there for a moment. I was overwhelmed with emotion that my daughter was growing up so quickly. We discussed what this meant and what she would need to do going forward. Her cycle produced a dark brown blood discharge on days one through three. On the fourth day there was a slight pink bloody discharge, but it was still mostly brown. She never experienced any real red menstrual blood flow during her first cycle. Her cycle lasted for 7 days.

Brett says:

I got my first period after most of my friends had, and I had had a lot of previous education about what to expect. Especially with an OB-GYN as a mother, I had a supply of pads and tampons, and when I first got my period I just proceeded to use a pad and inform my mom of the development. Even despite the fact that my mother was an OB-GYN and I had discussed the menstrual cycle in school, it was with my older brother's girlfriend that I talked about the more embarrassing aspects of getting my period. Having an older teenager to talk to was really helpful and helped me get past the seemingly awkward issues that accompany getting your period for the first time. However, it was also very important for me that I was able to tell my mom that I got my period without feeling self-conscious.

10. When should I expect my daughter to have her first period?

Half of all girls within the United States experience their first **period** before their 13th birthday. However, it's not terribly unusual to find a girl who began menstruating when she was as young as 9 or as old as 17.

In order to put the age issue into perspective, the following statistics may be helpful: 10% of girls **menstruate** by the time they're 11 years old; 90% of girls menstruate by the time they turn 14; and 98% of 15-year-old girls menstruate. If your daughter falls outside this age range, she should be examined by a pediatrician, just to make sure she doesn't have a medical problem.

Research has shown that African-American girls typically menstruate at the earliest age, followed by Hispanic girls and then non-Hispanic White girls. (Interestingly, there aren't any particularly reliable

Period

Refers to the periodic bleeding that occurs monthly from the uterus. Also known as the menstrual cycle.

10% of girls menstruate by the time they're 11 years old; 90% of girls menstruate by the time they turn 14; and 98% of 15-year-old girls menstruate.

Menstruate

The release of the menstrual blood from the uterus and out of the vagina.

13

Menstrual flow

The amount of blood that exits the vagina during a menstrual cycle.

Anemia

A medical condition characterized by a low blood count, which means that the patient does not have enough red blood cells. Anemia is sometimes seen in females who experience heavy menstrual bleeding. Symptoms often include fatigue and pale skin, and may include shortness of breath and chest pain.

Polycystic ovarian syndrome

A common hormonal disorder seen in young women and female adolescents that involves a variety of symptoms. Classic symptoms include infrequent menstrual cycles, acne, excessive hair growth, obesity, and a cystic appearance of the ovaries on sonograms.

Spotting

A very light, scanty amount of bleeding from the vagina that can be bright red or dark brown in color. Often this kind of bleeding is seen at the very beginning or the very end of a woman's menstrual cycle.

statistics for other ethnic groups.) Your doctor will take these facts into consideration when evaluating your daughter's health.

11. What is an average menstrual flow?

As with adult females, the average length of **menstrual flow** for adolescent girls is 7 days or less. During her period, your daughter is likely to use between three and six pads or tampons per day. If her flow is significantly above this amount, you should contact your pediatrician.

For example, a heavy flow requiring changes of menstrual products every 1 to 2 hours is excessive, especially if the flow lasts longer than 7 days. Not only could this condition lead to **anemia**, light-headedness, or even fainting, it could also be a sign of **polycystic ovarian syndrome**, anorexia, tumors, other chronic illnesses, or side effects from medication, so have it checked out.

12. How does an adolescent girl's period differ from that of an adult woman?

A girl's first period may be a brighter red than what you're used to seeing, and it likely will consist of a smaller amount of blood. In fact, your daughter's first period may really be nothing more than some **spotting**. But as her menstrual cycle continues, her periods are likely to become more pronounced and may remain irregular the first year.

13. Can my daughter become pregnant as soon as she starts menstruating?

For the first year or so after your daughter begins menstruating, she likely will not be ovulating. However, it's important to note that no girl who has just started having periods should rely on this fact in the expectation that she won't become pregnant if she has **sexual intercourse**. Rather, she needs to be mindful of the **safe-sex** precautions I spell out in other parts of this book.

14. How frequently will my daughter have periods?

Once your daughter's menstrual cycle becomes more regular, she should expect to have a period every 25 to 30 days. However, it's not uncommon for girls to have periods as frequently as every 21 days, or as spread out as every 45 days.

The time lapse between periods is highly dependent upon genetics, stress, and weight. You should also know that there are many documented cases where girls have essentially stopped having periods during times of grueling physical exertion, such as long-term training to run in marathons, or if they are anorexic. The American College of Obstetricians and Gynecologists recommends that adolescent females seek a medical evaluation if they have irregular menstrual cycles that occur less than every 90 days.

15. When will my daughter enter puberty?

Interestingly, there are a number of factors that can influence when a girl enters puberty. Of course, as we've seen, genetics plays a very important role. However, there are other variables as well, some of which are rather surprising. For instance, not only does nutrition have an impact on when a girl first begins menstruating, but so too does the altitude at which the girl lives, how close she lives to the equator, and how heavy she is; some researchers even claim it can be affected by whether there is a father-figure in the household.

Sexual intercourse

The insertion of the erect male penis into the female vagina.

Safe sex

Sexual activity that incorporates the use of birth control and condoms to minimize the risk of pregnancy and transmission of sexually transmitted infections.

Once your daughter's menstrual cycle becomes more regular, she should expect to have a period every 25 to 30 days.

Menstruation

Prostaglandins

A group of naturally occurring hormonal substances that have a widespread effect on the human body. One type of prostaglandin is produced by the uterus and causes contractions of the uterine muscle. High levels of prostaglandin have been associated with painful menstrual cramps.

Uterus

A hollow, pear-shaped organ in the pelvis where a developing fetus grows. The lower part is attached to the cervix. The lining of the uterus sheds monthly as the menstrual period.

Naprosyn

A common over-the-counter, antiprostaglandin product that is used for menstrual cramps, headaches, and other pains. One example is Aleve.

Antiprostaglandins

Medications that counteract the effects of prostaglandins. Ibuprofen and naprosyn are examples of over-the-counter antiprostaglandins.

In general, during the past few decades there has been a noticeable decrease in the age at which girls in the United States enter puberty. Some people believe that this is a direct result of the hormones that are administered to cows. Their concern is that these hormones eventually end up in the cows' milk, and then, in turn, they end up in our daughters' bodies when they drink this milk. This hypothesis has been hotly debated over the years, but as of now, it is not generally accepted by the medical community. The more accepted theory regarding the declining age for the onset of periods relates to the increased prevalence of childhood obesity. Simply stated, the heavier the adolescent girl, the earlier she will menstruate.

16. What symptoms will my daughter experience during her periods?

Many girls and women notice a change in their bowel habits around the time of their period. This is caused by **prostaglandins**, which are hormones released by the **uterus** during a menstrual cycle. These prostaglandins can cause nausea, intestinal cramping, and diarrhea. These unpleasant symptoms can occur to such a degree that otherwise healthy women and girls find it necessary to stay home from work or school during "that time of the month."

When my patients tell me they're experiencing these problems, I recommend that they take ibuprofen or **Naprosyn**. These medications are known as **antiprostaglandins**. As such, they can alleviate the nausea, cramping, and diarrhea. Similarly, oral **contraceptives** can greatly reduce these symptoms because they, too, have an antiprostaglandin effect.

Donna says:

During my daughter's menstrual cycle she experienced some discomfort in her breasts. She indicated that they were tender to the touch. She also had some cramping. I gave her some ibuprofen for the discomfort and that took care of it. Her stomach seems to be upset with certain foods during her cycle, and she needs more rest.

Brett says:

Usually, my period is only accompanied by cramps. Sometimes, these cramps are quick and over in a short time, but sometimes they can be very painful and it is hard to concentrate in school. It is really important that if you to tend to get these bad symptoms to know how to deal with them. When my cramps are at their worst, I tend to take Advil, which alleviates the majority of the pain in about 20 minutes. However, when I have only minor symptoms, such as bloating, minor cardio exercise like a jog for only 15 minutes, can really help.

17. What body changes accompany menstruation?

Once your daughter's menstrual cycle begins, she's going to notice some other bodily changes as well. Because of a rise in estrogen levels, which stimulates the vaginal tissue and the glands in the **vagina,** she is going to experience more secretions and lubrication. In fact, a small amount of non-odorous **vaginal discharge** is normal.

During this time frame, a girl's vagina also becomes colonized by "good" bacteria. These are known as **lactobacillus bacteria,** and they are essential in balancing the environment in the vagina and warding off infections.

Menstruation

Contraceptives

A general term that encompasses methods, medications, and devices to prevent pregnancy.

Vagina

The muscular, tube-like organ that extends from the uterus and cervix to the outside of the body. The opening is located in between the urethra and the anus. It is lined with glands that produce mucous secretions.

Vaginal discharge

A mucus-like substance coming from the vagina. A small amount of non-odorous discharge can be normal. A large amount of discharge accompanied by itching, odor, or unusual color can indicate an infection.

Lactobacillus bacteria

The "good" bacteria found in the vagina that are responsible for maintaining a normal vaginal environment. These bacteria help fight off bad bacteria that cause vaginal and urinary tract infections.

18. Why are bladder infections more common in younger girls?

Bladder infection

A common infection in women that occurs when bacteria gain entry into the bladder.

Urethra

The short tube that opens just in front of the vagina. It carries urine from the bladder to the outside.

Prior to puberty, girls are more susceptible to **bladder infections**. This is because the **urethra** (which is the opening to the bladder) is in such close proximity to the rectum. Bacteria from the rectum are what cause the vast majority of bladder infections in girls. (That's why young girls should be taught to wipe from front to back after they have a bowel movement.) It is the introduction of estrogen that begins the process of strengthening the wall between the vagina and bladder, replacing the "bad" bacteria with the "good" bacteria, and building up the tissue of the urethra, which then becomes a stronger barrier and helps prevent the remaining "bad" bacteria from entering the bladder. (Yes, sometimes our bodies seem to serve as the backdrop for a superheroes cartoon.)

19. Why are preventive health visits important?

The American Academy of Pediatrics and the American College of Obstetricians and Gynecologists both recommend routine preventive health visits for adolescent girls.

The American Academy of Pediatrics and the American College of Obstetricians and Gynecologists both recommend routine preventive health visits for adolescent girls. I strongly encourage you to follow their guidance. These visits not only provide an opportunity for a doctor to evaluate your daughter's health, but they also provide both you and your daughter with an opportunity to answer any questions you may have.

These check-ups can be part of a routine appointment with a family doctor. Similarly, a pediatrician can evaluate your daughter's health, and they typically are an excellent source of information. As an alternative, you should feel free to schedule an appointment for your daughter with a **gynecologist**. I can assure you that in most cases there will be no need for the gynecologist to conduct a **pelvic exam**.

20. What menstrual issues should prompt me to take my daughter to a doctor?

In addition to routine preventive health visits, there are certain signs related to menstruation that should prompt you to contact a doctor about your daughter's health. Specifically, you should schedule an appointment if your daughter's menstrual period:

- has not started within 3 years of her breast development;
- has not started by age 13 and there are no other signs of the onset of puberty;
- has not started by age 14 and she is experiencing excessive hair growth on her body;
- has not started by age 14 and you suspect that she is engaging in excessive exercise or may have an eating disorder:
- has not started by age 15;
- became regular, but then became noticeably irregular;
- occurs more frequently than every 21 days or less frequently than every 45 days;
- occurs more than 90 days apart, even for just 1 cycle;
- lasts more than 7 days;
- requires frequent pad or tampon changes (such as soaking more than one pad or tampon every 1 to 2 hours).

In many cases, even with these signs and symptoms, a doctor will conclude that an adolescent girl is just fine. But in other cases, medical treatment will be required. That's why medical evaluations are so helpful. They're indispensable to us as we fulfill our sacred responsibility as mothers.

Gynecologist

A medical doctor who specializes in the care of women and the treatment of diseases that affect their sexual organs.

Pelvic exam

An examination of the female reproductive organs. This exam can include an external inspection of the genital region, a speculum exam of the vagina and cervix, and/or a manual exam of the internal genital organs, i.e., the uterus and cervix.

Menstruation

PART THREE

Sanitary Pads and Tampons

What should my daughter know about sanitary pads?

When should my daughter use tampons?

What is my daughter's risk of getting TSS and how can she avoid it?

More . . .

One topic that always generates a lot of questions from mothers involves when and if a newly menstruating girl should switch from **sanitary pads** to tampons. Whether a Mom asks me during her own gynecological exam, or whether I get pulled aside by a parent at my children's elementary school, the questions are usually the same. When should my daughter start using tampons? How long can she leave one in? Can she wear it overnight? Which one is best? What about Toxic Shock Syndrome? Is there a book to tell her how to use one?

The first thing I tell moms is that until an adolescent girl is ready to use a tampon, it's fruitless to try to force her to. We probably all remember when we made that transition from pads to tampons—you had to be ready. In fact, I have grown patients who still will not use tampons for one reason or another, and that's fine. It's their personal choice. The same principle holds true with your daughter.

21. What should my daughter know about sanitary pads?

Sanitary pads are the mainstay for adolescent girls as they adjust to the new phenomenon of menstruating. As I think back to the days when you had to fiddle with the old sanitary napkin belt and the bulky, leaky pads of the 1970s, I realize just how much easier girls have it now. Pads nowadays are more absorbent, more comfortable, and have better features such as side wings and increased length to prevent leakage.

These aren't the only changes when it comes to sanitary pads. When disposable pads first became available, in many stores women placed their money in a box and then took a package of sanitary napkins from the counter so that they wouldn't have to undergo the

Sanitary pads

A pad of absorbent material worn to absorb menstrual blood.

embarrassment of dealing with the male sales clerk. But today, you're likely to end up viewing a multitude of commercials for sanitary pads while you're just trying to watch a little TV with your teenaged son.

Donna says:

When my daughter started her menstrual cycle, she and I discussed what sanitary products are and how to use them. Given my daughter's young age of 11 years old when she started, we decided to start off using sanitary pads. We didn't think tampons would be appropriate at her age. We discussed what the different size pads were to ensure she understood what light, medium, and heavy flow pads were used for and how to choose the right one for her cycle. We also discussed panty liners and pads with wings.

On day one her menstrual bleeding was light. I explained to her you can use a light to medium size pad for protection. As her menstrual bleeding increases, she will need to decide what sanitary pad will give her the right absorbent protection. We also discussed personal hygiene. I told her it is very important to keep yourself clean and replace your sanitary pad. Depending on her menstrual bleeding she will need to change her pad anywhere from 4 to 5 times a day to ensure there is no leaking and no menstrual odor, which can happen during her cycle.

22. What are the different types of sanitary pads?

Popular disposable sanitary pads are made mostly of wood cellulose fiber with an outer cover of moisture-proof plastic. There are several different types.

Panty Liner—a very thin pad designed to absorb a daily vaginal discharge, light menstrual flow, "spotting," slight urinary incontinence, or for use as a backup when a tampon is being used

Ultra-thin—a very compact pad which typically is as absorbent as a regular or maxi/super pad, but with less bulk

Regular—a middle-range absorbency pad

Maxi/Super—a highly absorbent pad that is useful for the start of a menstrual cycle when menstruation is often heaviest

Night—a highly absorbent pad that is also longer, thereby offering more protection while the wearer is lying down

Maternity—a long, very absorbent pad designed to absorb the bleeding that occurs after childbirth

Thong Panty Liner—a pad designed especially to fit thong underwear

When you're shopping for pads with your daughter, you'll probably end up buying a few different types to see which one works best for her. Because I see many young, as well as older, women with symptoms of skin irritation on their bottoms, I always recommend to my patients that they buy products that are white (no dyes) and unscented (no perfumes) to avoid as many irritants as possible.

And although it may seem obvious, you need to explain to your daughter why it's important not to attempt to flush a sanitary pad down the toilet. Tell her that although it may seem embarrassing to have someone notice that you just disposed of a sanitary pad in the trash, it is far more embarrassing to make people tiptoe through overflowing water because you threw a used sanitary pad in the toilet.

Donna says:

I shared with my daughter that there are different types of sanitary pads with different absorbency. We discussed what a panty liner was and when they are to be used. We discussed when to use medium to heavy pads. I told her that overnight pads can be worn for additional protection while she is sleeping. I told her that these pads come with or without wings. Wings are to hold the sanitary pad in place. Pads come in lightly scented or perfume free. I explained to her since she has sensitive skin, perfume free would be better for her.

23. What are reusable menstrual pads?

One product that seems to be gaining increased attention is reusable menstrual pads. These are washable, highly-absorbent cloths that are usually secured by wings around the underwear. In many ways they are a modern version of what was used by women in "the old days" during their menstrual cycles. (In fact, it's from this practice that the demeaning and archaic phrase "on the rag" comes from.)

Although relatively few women use reusable menstrual pads, they do have certain advantages:

* They are allergen-free, chemical-free, and perfume-free and are thus less likely to cause irritation and contact dermatitis on the **vulva** and the vagina, and they are generally more comfortable for women with sensitive skin.
* They are less expensive than disposable pads over the long term.
* They carry less menstrual odor and are more breathable.

Vulva

The external female genital organs that include the labia majora, labia minora, clitoris, Bartholins glands, and the opening to the vagina (vestibule).

- They are environmentally friendly because they are made of natural materials rather than plastic and do not contribute to growing landfill problems.

Reusable pads do have disadvantages, however. For instance:

- They are more time consuming due to the need to wash and dry them.
- Washing them is not particularly easy because the water with the menstrual blood needs to be disposed of properly.
- If the user has a **yeast infection** the pad must be sanitized in order to prevent re-infection.
- Their initial cost is higher, although over time they become more economical.

Reusable menstrual pads are certainly not for everyone, but they are worth considering if they fit your lifestyle.

24. When should my daughter use tampons?

After using sanitary pads for a while, it's likely that your daughter will tell you one day that she'd like to try **tampons**. That means it's time for you to go to the store and stare at the many options on the shelf. (And when I say "you," I mean that in the singular rather than the plural form. Unless you're willing to travel to a different state and perform your task in disguise, don't count on your adolescent daughter being willing to stand in a store aisle next to you as you both publicly survey the menstrual products they have available.)

25. What are the different types of tampons?

The Food and Drug Administration now regulates tampon absorbency, which is defined as the rate at which a

Yeast infection

One of the most common vaginal infections among women. This infection is not sexually transmitted. Yeast is commonly present in the vagina in very small amounts. A change in the balance of the vaginal flora often caused by taking an antibiotic will cause the yeast to overgrow and symptoms of itching and discharge can occur.

Tampon

A plug of absorbent material placed in the vagina to prevent menstrual blood from coming out.

tampon soaks up menstrual blood. Absorbency is measured in grams of fluid, and you will find absorbency ratings on all tampon boxes. Specifically, the following tampons are readily available:

- Light or Junior Absorbency: 6 grams of blood or less. This tampon is good for the end of a woman's period when she has the lightest flow.
- Regular Absorbency: 6 to 9 grams of blood. As the name suggests, this tampon is good for many women on most days of their periods.
- Super Absorbency: 9 to 12 grams of blood. This tampon will provide the extra absorption that some women need on their first 1 to 2 days of heavier bleeding.
- Super-Plus Absorbency: 12 to 15 grams of blood. Some women experience especially heavy bleeding on their period and may require this tampon.
- Ultra-Absorbency: 15 to 18 grams of blood. Most women will never need to use this tampon. If this tampon is necessary, a visit to the gynecologist may be wise in order to evaluate the cause of this extremely heavy menstruation.

26. How can my daughter choose the right tampon?

The type of tampon that is right for your daughter depends on her menstrual flow. Simply stated, she should match the absorbency of the tampon to her flow. If she has a light flow, then she should try the junior or regular tampon. If her tampon is completely soaked before 4 hours, she should try one with higher absorbency.

However, you should caution your daughter that if a tampon is too absorbent for her flow, vaginal dryness

Absorbency is measured in grams of fluid, and you will find absorbency ratings on all tampon boxes.

Sanitary Pads and Tampons

Toxic Shock Syndrome (TSS)

A rare and potentially lethal illness caused by toxins excreted from bacteria. Historically linked to tampon use, Toxic Shock Syndrome can occur anytime these toxins have an opportunity to gain access into the human body. Symptoms include fever, a drop in blood pressure, rash, peeling of skin from palms and soles, nausea and vomiting, liver inflammation, renal failure, low blood platelets, and confusion.

Staph bacteria

A common type of bacteria normally found on skin surfaces that can cause infections. The staphylococcus aureus bacteria can produce a toxin that is the cause of Toxic Shock Syndrome.

Toxin

A poisonous product of animal and plant cells or bacteria that causes tissue damage and antibody formation.

and even vaginal ulcerations can occur. If a tampon is dry and hard to remove, shreds, or doesn't need to be changed for many hours, she should switch to a less absorbent tampon. Why is this important? Because research suggests that the risk of Toxic Shock Syndrome may increase with tampon absorbency. However, please note this doesn't mean your daughter should shy away from using higher absorbency tampons if she really needs them.

27. What is Toxic Shock Syndrome?

Toxic Shock Syndrome (or TSS) is a rare but potentially life-threatening illness. Researchers believe it is caused by an infection resulting from certain staph and strep bacteria that often exist even in a healthy woman's vagina. The exact process is unknown, but it's thought that these bacteria multiply in the presence of a blood-soaked tampon. It's actually not the bacteria that cause the TSS directly. Rather, it's the toxins that the bacteria produce that do the harm.

It's important to note that **staph bacteria** are very common. We all have them on our skin and inside our noses. Usually they are harmless, but if they gain access to the bloodstream or deeper tissue, they can cause a serious infection.

For TSS to occur, certain strains of the bacteria have to overpopulate and produce large amounts of **toxin**. This toxin then has to gain access to the bloodstream. One generally accepted theory is that super-absorbent tampons that are left in the vagina for extended periods of time can encourage growth of the bacteria. And importantly, these super-absorbent tampons can also adhere to the vaginal wall if they are dry and the menstrual flow is light, thereby causing tiny abrasions when removed.

These abrasions then provide access to deeper tissue or to the bloodstream for the bacteria and toxins.

28. What are the symptoms of TSS?

The symptoms of TSS include fever, vomiting, dizziness, diarrhea, fainting, a sunburn-like rash, muscle aches, sore throat, headache, joint pain, red eyes, and sensitivity to light. As the illness progresses, TSS can also lead to mental confusion, kidney failure, a drop in blood pressure, and collapse. One to two weeks after the initial symptoms, peeling patches of skin on the palms and soles can occur.

These symptoms typically appear during a woman's period or a few days after. If a woman suspects she has TSS, she should remove her tampon immediately and call her doctor or go to the emergency room for immediate evaluation. Treatment requires hospital admission for intravenous antibiotics to kill the bacteria, intravenous fluids to treat the low blood pressure and dehydration, and observation and treatment for signs of kidney failure. With appropriate treatment, most patients will recover in 2 to 3 weeks.

29. What is my daughter's risk of getting TSS and how can she avoid it?

Younger females, such as those under 30, may be at a higher risk for TSS because they have not yet formed **antibodies** to the staph toxin. Therefore, it's important for you and your daughter to be vigilant for TSS. However, it's also important to know that there now are actually very few TSS cases reported each year.

Toxic Shock Syndrome became a hot topic in 1980 when 813 cases of menstrual-related cases of TSS—and

The symptoms of TSS include fever, vomiting, dizziness, diarrhea, fainting, a sunburn-like rash, muscle aches, sore throat, headache, joint pain, red eyes, and sensitivity to light.

Antibodies

Microscopic particles in the body that fight infection. Antibodies are manufactured by the body in response to vaccinations. For example, the HPV vaccines promote antibody production to help fight off an HPV infection.

38 deaths—were reported. Research ended up showing that use of a specific type of tampon that is no longer on the market put women at a higher risk of TSS than use of other tampons. This tampon was made with a new combination of materials including polyester foam and a highly absorbent cellulose that enhanced absorption. Although not all TSS cases occurred in women who used this specific type of tampon, it clearly played an important role. Therefore, it was removed from the market, along with other new, highly absorbent tampons of similar substances.

Because of the discontinued use of these types of tampons, as well as the Food and Drug Administration's regulation of tampon materials and absorbency, there has been a dramatic drop in the number of TSS cases. In 1997, only six cases were confirmed, and in 1998, only three cases. Nevertheless, the FDA recommends that women take the following steps to avoid tampon problems:

- Follow the package directions for insertion;
- Choose the lowest absorbency that will handle your menstrual flow;
- Change your tampon at least every 4 to 8 hours;
- Consider alternating pads with tampons;
- Don't use tampons between periods; and
- Know the warning signs of Toxic Shock Syndrome.

I would add the following recommendations:

- Keep your tampon clean by keeping it in its wrapper until you're ready to use it. A small carrying case is helpful. It doesn't have to look like a tampon container.
- Wear sanitary pads at night, if possible. If the flow is heavy and you have to change during the night,

it's okay to use a tampon for up to 8 hours so that your sleep is not interrupted.

In my 20 years of practice, I have seen only one case of Toxic Shock Syndrome. However, every couple of months I see at least one patient who has forgotten that she inserted a tampon a few days, or even a few weeks, earlier. The patient invariably comes in because she has noticed a really bad odor coming from her vagina. A *really* bad odor. And yet, none of these patients has ever developed any health problems from the forgotten tampon. Needless to say, however, I strongly encourage all of my patients to keep track of their tampon use. Not only does it reduce the risk of TSS, it also reduces the risk of vaginitis and pelvic infections.

30. What myths about tampons are circulating on the Internet?

When your daughter starts using tampons, she'll probably rely on the Internet or her friends to get information about them. You should know that tall tales abound when it comes to tampons, and questionable Web sites often add unfounded, unproven, and just plain wrong information. Therefore, it's important for you to be able to set the record straight. In doing so, you should remember the following facts to combat common, but completely silly, rumors:

1. Tampons **CANNOT** be lost forever in a woman's body. A tampon remains in the vagina no matter what. It cannot migrate anywhere else.
2. Tampons do **NOT** cause AIDS.
3. Manufacturers do **NOT** add asbestos or other materials to tampons to cause an increase in menstrual bleeding, which then boosts sales.

4. Tampons do **NOT** contain hazardous levels of dioxins which are cancer-causing agents and which are claimed to be produced through the tampon bleaching process. (The bleaching process is designed to clean and purify the raw materials used in tampons. In conjunction with the Environmental Protection Agency, tampon manufacturers tested their products for dioxin. The levels of dioxin in tampons ranged from undetectable to 1 part in 3 trillion, far below the level that occurs through daily environmental exposure and considerably below the level the FDA believes would put consumers at risk.)

5. Tampon use does **NOT** affect virginity.

31. Are there helpful tips for inserting tampons?

Now that you know all of this information about tampons, it's time to tell you the secret to effortlessly inserting tampons so that you can pass it along to your daughter.

But guess what? The secret is that there really is no secret. We gynecologists don't have any special insights or methods that we learned in medical school or elsewhere. (Sorry about that.) However, the tips and steps listed below can be quite helpful to you and your daughter.

- First, your daughter should read the instructions in the tampon package. The pictures that accompany the directions can be particularly helpful.
- You should tactfully ask your daughter whether she wants help inserting a tampon for the first time. It's her decision.

- Your daughter should try her first tampon on one of the days that her menstrual flow is the heaviest. This helps to ensure that dryness is not an issue during insertion or removal.
- Your daughter should start out using "slim" or "slender" tampons because they tend to be more comfortable. Also, it would probably be wise for her to choose a tampon with a rounded, smooth applicator because they typically are more comfortable than applicators with blunt ends.
- She may want to apply a small amount of lubrication such as K-Y Jelly to the applicator tip because it can help ease the insertion.
- Your daughter should find a position that is comfortable for her to insert the tampon. Most women insert a tampon while sitting on the toilet, but other women, especially adolescents, may find it's easier if they remain standing in the bathroom and place one foot up on the toilet seat.
- Your daughter should relax as she inserts the tampon. Tensing the vaginal muscles causes resistance to the tampon, thereby making insertion more uncomfortable.
- She should hold the applicator between her thumb and her middle finger. Her index finger should be kept free so that she can push in the tampon.
- Using her other hand, she should separate the **labia** (lips) of her vagina and insert the tampon applicator into the vaginal opening.
- Some adolescents find that a small hand mirror is initially helpful in locating the vaginal opening.
- Using her index finger, she should push the tampon all the way in while holding the applicator steady with her thumb and forefinger.
- She should then remove the applicator, being careful not to pull on the tampon string.

Labia

The folds of tissue on the vulva. There are two sets of labia, the labia majora (outer) and the labia minora (inner).

- Your daughter can remove the tampon at any time simply by pulling on the string.

It's important for your daughter to know that once the tampon is inserted she shouldn't feel it or even sense that it's there. If it's constantly making its presence known, it may be positioned incorrectly or not be inserted far enough. The best thing to do in that case is to remove the tampon and try again with a new one. Remind your daughter that practice makes perfect with tampon use, and with time it will become a comfortable routine—during a rather uncomfortable time of the month.

PART FOUR

Hygiene

Should my adolescent daughter use antiperspirants
or deodorants?

Why is my daughter starting to suffer from acne?

As a mother of a daughter entering puberty,
what skin care advice can I give her?

More . . .

Once your daughter reaches puberty, you can kiss good-bye those easy days of her childhood when all you had to do to bathe her was occasionally dip her in the tub and quickly shampoo her hair. Much to your dismay in social settings, once puberty strikes you will likely notice that your daughter frequently develops body odor that can be quite strong. (And interestingly, you also may discover that she is quite oblivious to the smell.)

32. What can be done to reduce body odor?

The source of your daughter's body odor is her skin glands, especially under her arms. Beginning around the time they're 8 years old, girls produce more sweat in this area. Initially, human sweat is odorless. (Honest!) But when it becomes mixed with the bacteria that are normally present on a person's skin, and then you add in some body heat, watch out. The funky odor begins.

Once this biological process begins for your daughter, she may need to begin bathing daily in order to reduce the amount of bacteria on her skin. This doesn't need to be an elaborate process of soaking in bubble bath and scrubbing her skin raw. (In fact, both of these steps would do more harm than good to her body.) Rather, a quick rinse in the shower with a mild soap on a regular basis should do the trick.

Another step you can take to help your daughter in this embarrassing situation is to buy her loose-fitting clothing made of natural fibers. These types of clothes allow air to circulate around your daughter's body and let her sweat evaporate. And needless to say, she shouldn't wear sweaty clothes two days in a row.

If regular showering and the appropriate clothing don't fully address the problem, you may want to consider having your daughter use **antibacterial** soap. Also, you should take a look at her diet. As we all know as adults, people can take a shower every day and wear only freshly laundered clothes, but if they eat food with lots of garlic, onions, and spices, they're undoubtedly going to produce a noticeable body odor. (And, undoubtedly, they'll end up standing right next to you on a crowded elevator.)

33. Should my adolescent daughter use antiperspirants or deodorants?

What if all these measures *still* don't affect that lingering, ripe cloud that hovers over your daughter? What next? Should you turn to antiperspirants and deodorants? Perhaps you've heard rumors about the potential link between the use of deodorants and antiperspirants and the incidence of breast cancer in women. Is this true? Would you be harming your daughter by exposing her to hazardous chemicals for a trivial reason?

First, let's start with some definitions. **Deodorants** are substances that are applied under a person's arms for the purpose of reducing body odor by killing bacteria that would otherwise interact with the person's sweat. Deodorants are often alcohol-based because it's very effective at killing bacteria.

Antiperspirants are a little different than deodorants. These substances are designed to reduce or stop a person from sweating in the first place. Antiperspirants typically work by plugging the sweat glands with an aluminum-based complex.

In the 1990s, concerns arose that perhaps the aluminum in antiperspirants and the preservatives (called **parabens**)

Antibacterial

The ability to fight off or destroy bacteria.

Hygiene

Deodorants

Products sold over-the-counter that are used to decrease body odor arising from sweat under a person's arms. Deodorants contain substances such as alcohol that kill odor-producing skin bacteria. They may be combined with antiperspirants that decrease sweat production.

Antiperspirants

Chemicals typically used to block secretion of sweat from sweat glands under a person's arms.

Parabens

Chemical preservatives found in many cosmetic products and deodorants.

in deodorants caused breast cancer. The prevailing theory behind this concern was that these substances could cause cancer by preventing people from sweating out the toxins in their bodies. These toxins, the theory went, would then spread via the **lymph nodes** and cause cancer.

Lymph nodes

Small bean-like structures that contain white blood cells and help fight infection. They are scattered throughout the body.

Further, one large study conducted in 2003 and involving 800 women specifically found no link between the use of antiperspirants or deodorants and an increased incidence of breast cancer.

To date, this theory regarding the use of antiperspirants and deodorants has not been supported by solid evidence. In fact, the National Cancer Institute has officially stated that these claims are "largely unsubstantiated by scientific research." Further, one large study conducted in 2003 and involving 800 women specifically found no link between the use of antiperspirants or deodorants and an increased incidence of breast cancer.

Nevertheless, research continues in this area. One hypothesis is that aluminum and parabens could have a mild estrogen-like effect when they work their way into a woman's body. Scientists are studying whether this is true, and if so, whether it would pose a cancer risk.

If you want to be cautious, you may want to have your daughter try a natural deodorant. These products are readily available and do not contain aluminum or parabens. However, they also may not be as effective for your daughter. If that's the case, then your daughter may want to try a judicious amount of a standard deodorant or antiperspirant. (Or, you simply may want to ensure that she always stands downwind from you.)

34. Why is my daughter starting to suffer from acne?

Few things cause more stress and embarrassment for adolescent girls than pimples and blemishes on their faces. Acne affects almost 90% of teenagers and is brought on by the rise in androgens, or male-like hormones, that occurs with puberty. There are many misconceptions about acne and what causes it. Contrary to popular belief, foods like French fries, soda, pizza, and chocolate do not cause acne. And while it is obviously a good idea for your daughter to wash her face, overzealous, frequent scrubbing with strong soap will do more harm than good. The irritation caused to the skin may actually encourage the formation of acne.

Acne affects almost 90% of teenagers and is brought on by the rise in androgens, or male-like hormones, that occurs with puberty.

Hygiene

35. As a mother of a daughter entering puberty, what skin care advice can I give her?

Your daughter should wash her face with a gentle cleanser no more than twice a day. She should use non-alcohol based cleansers that contain alpha-hydroxy acid or beta-hydroxy acid (salicylic acid) because these will gently exfoliate the skin. After washing, an over-the-counter product containing benzoyl peroxide should be used to kill the bacteria causing the acne. "Popping" pimples is a very bad idea because it can force bacteria deeper into the skin and cause scarring. Minimizing makeup and using only oil-free, water-based products will be helpful too.

If these measures don't clear up the acne, the next step is to have your daughter see a doctor and be evaluated for the need to use a stronger medicine or antibiotic. (Interestingly, the birth control pill can be very helpful in controlling acne. The pills cause a decrease in the circulating androgen levels and thus reduce the primary cause of acne.)

Brett says:

Before going to extreme measures with acne medication, it is really important to just wash your face and apply lotion and sunscreen. Find good face washes, lotions, and sunscreens for sale that are designed for sensitive skin. I began to see a dermatologist in seventh grade and used a combination of products until I found ones that worked the best. I alternate between Tazorac® and Epiduo™, and I use Keflex as an oral medicine. It is really important to find products that won't dry out your skin and will give you the best results.

36. What causes dermatitis in the genital area?

In my medical practice, I see more than my fair share of irritated bottoms. (That's part of the glamorous life of a gynecologist.) A significant portion of these cases is caused by one of two types of contact dermatitis. Unfortunately, this problem affects the **genital** region just like any other part of the body.

Irritant contact **dermatitis** is caused by repeated exposure to a caustic or physically irritating substance such as urine, feces, or soap residue. The primary causes include over-washing, use of creams with drying bases, the persistent wetness that can occur from menstruation, urine, or feces, and incomplete rinsing of clothing so that soap residue on underwear interacts on the skin when the woman perspires. Panty liners and **douches** are other causes of irritation.

Allergic contact dermatitis is an allergic reaction to something that touches your skin. The more common substances include neomycin, benzacaine, preservatives (parabens and propylene glycol), latex (condoms), chlorhexidine, nail polish, lanolin, and perfume. You will be surprised to find these ingredients in very commonly used over-the-counter products.

While there are so many wonderful-smelling bath salts, soaps, and body washes out there these days,

Genitals

A term that refers to a person's internal and external sexual organs.

Dermatitis

An irritation of the skin that can be caused by an infection or the use of a product such as a soap, lotion, or powder. The symptoms can include itching, burning, and general discomfort.

Douches

Liquids that are inserted in the vagina for the purpose of cleansing the vagina. These commonly contain vinegar and can be bought over-the-counter or made at home. Douching is not generally recommended by the medical community.

I advise my patients to stick to mild soaps that have no perfumes or additives. A good rule of thumb for you and your daughter to keep in mind is, "The better they smell, the worse they irritate."

I have seen young girls who need to urinate frequently and are evaluated for bladder infections. And yet, these symptoms completely cleared up when they simply stopped using fruity shampoos and yummy-smelling bubble baths. This was most likely because these soaps and shampoos had an irritant effect on their urinary areas. Therefore, I recommend to patients who are prone to skin irritation that they use **hypoallergenic** soaps available in most stores.

Although we live in a largely shower-oriented society, a soak in the bathtub with just warm water and mild soap is often just what the female genital area needs for cleansing and soothing. The soak seems to do a better job at rinsing away the bad bacteria in the vaginal area, and at calming irritated skin. Though everyone is in a rush today and showers are quick, a 10- or 15-minute bath on a periodic basis could do your daughter a lot of good.

37. Should my daughter be shaving and waxing?

One final hygiene topic involves shaving and waxing. (I'll cover this topic in greater depth in the chapter on body art.) Many adolescents feel the need to shave their legs, even before they hit middle school. Those with darker hair in particular tend to feel that their leg hair or underarm hair is very noticeable and, therefore, a source of embarrassment. As long as your daughter is instructed in how to shave and the use of a safety razor, there shouldn't be a problem.

Hypoallergenic
A product that has a low likelihood of causing an allergic reaction.

A soak in the bathtub with just warm water and mild soap is often just what the female genital area needs for cleansing and soothing.

Shaving and waxing of the pubic region is a little different. I see many young women with irritation and itchiness in the pubic area caused by shaving. An exam often shows that they have ingrown hairs and red bumps caused by the inflammation of their hair follicles. Therefore, you may want to recommend to your daughter that if she really wants to reduce the amount of her pubic hair, she should keep it limited to simple trimming with an appropriate pair of scissors.

Kama says:

If you will read the directions on the back of your cream hair remover, you may find a caution statement that reads, in part "Do not use on recently tweezed or shaved areas." There may be no mention of recently waxed areas. Recently waxed areas are hypersensitive and the skin contains tiny pockets where the hair shafts used to reside. Learn from others' mistakes is a wonderful adage. Therefore, allow me. Do NOT use cream hair remover on recently waxed skin or you will achieve a chemical burn like . . . you read about.

PART FIVE

Your Daughter's First Visit to a Gynecologist

What will happen at my daughter's first
visit to the gynecologist?

Many of my patients ask me when they should bring their daughters in to see me for their first gynecological visit. As with so many other facets of life, the real answer is, "It depends."

The American College of Obstetricians and Gynecologists (ACOG) recommends that adolescent girls make their first visit to a gynecologist for screening and preventive counseling between the ages of 13 and 15. The content of this visit will vary with the individual patient because it will depend on the girl's needs and her physical and emotional development. However, you and your daughter should know that a pelvic exam will NOT be included as part of the visit except in those rare instances where the doctor believes it's really needed.

38. What will happen at my daughter's first visit to the gynecologist?

ACOG recommends that doctors perform the following procedures when an adolescent female between the ages of 13 and 18 comes in for a visit:

- A detailed history and physical
- Chlamydia and gonorrhea testing if the patient is sexually active
- Testing for HIV, Hepatitis B and C, and syphilis if the doctor believes it's warranted
- A discussion of nutrition, the menstrual cycle, sexual activity and practices, depression, exercise, contraception, and STD prevention
- Immunizations:
  - Tetanus/Diphtheria/Polio vaccine once between the ages of 11 and 16
  - Hepatitis B vaccine (if the patient was not vaccinated previously)
  - Human Papillomavirus (HPV) vaccine

○ Meningococcal conjugate vaccine before entry into high school (if the patient was not vaccinated previously)

Although these recommendations are clearly good ones, I rarely see any young women between the ages of 13 to 15 for a first preventive visit unless they have ongoing gynecological issues. I think this is largely due to the fact that most pediatricians do such an outstanding job of providing medical care and advice to their female adolescent patients.

Regardless of any age guidelines or any health issues, you should definitely bring your daughter to a gynecologist if you suspect she has become sexually active. Similarly, even if they are perfectly healthy and are not sexually active, I encourage all moms to bring in their daughters before they go off to college. As I noted earlier, if your daughter is not sexually active, she likely will not have to undergo a pelvic exam.

Regardless of any age guidelines or any health issues, you should definitely bring your daughter to a gynecologist if you suspect she has become sexually active.

The reason I choose college as a particular milestone is because it's a time of new independence for many girls and, with that, the freedom to make their own choices. This freedom often includes decisions about whether to become sexually active. Therefore, it's important for girls to hear the straightforward facts about the risks and hazards of sexual activity. (As you can see, paying for tuition isn't the only thing you have to worry about when your daughter goes off to college.)

When I meet with these young women, I talk to them candidly about sexually transmitted diseases and the options they have for **birth control**. I also give them information on the HPV vaccine (if they have not already been inoculated), and I start the vaccination series, which can then be finished at their schools. Even if they are not

Birth control
Various forms of medications, devices, or practices that help prevent pregnancy.

planning on becoming sexually active soon, I let them know that they can call me for birth control during the year in case they discover they need it. I have found that the student health centers at most universities are excellent about providing these services as well.

If a young woman still is not ready to come in for a visit by the time she's 18 and she is not sexually active, then I tell the mother that a pelvic exam and a **Pap smear** test are strongly recommended by age 21.

When I meet with young patients for the first time, they often want their mothers present for the interview and the exam. If a young patient is brought back to my office by herself, I always inquire whether her mother has accompanied her. If she has, then I make sure to ask the daughter what her preference is. Sometimes a girl is too embarrassed to ask that her mother accompany her; sometimes the patient definitely doesn't want her mother to be present; and sometimes the mother is simply trying to let the daughter make her own decision and do the visit by herself without asking the daughter what she actually would prefer. It's important to figure out the right approach for each patient.

If the mother is not present during the interview and exam, but she is present in the waiting room, I ask for the daughter's permission to bring her back at the end of the appointment to see if she has any questions. (Otherwise I usually get an awkward phone call from the chagrined mother later that day inquiring about the visit.) I always ask adolescent girls if I can speak with their mothers about their visit and the results of any tests I've conducted. In most cases the girls readily consent.

A mom's critical role in her daughter's life doesn't stop at the threshold of a doctor's office.

Pap smear

The sample of cells taken from the cervix during a speculum exam. Historically, the cells were smeared on a slide for interpretation in the lab. These days, the cells are released into a vial with liquid, cleansed, and then interpreted.

PART SIX

Sexually Transmitted Diseases

How important are condoms in preventing STDs?

How common are STD infections?

What is genital herpes?

More . . .

Did you know that approximately 85% of females will have some type of sexual contact (vaginal, oral, or anal) either with a male or another female by the time they're 19 years old? Did you know that almost one-third of ninth-grade girls have had sexual intercourse? Did you know that more than 60% of twelfth-grade girls have had sexual intercourse?

Have I alarmed you yet?

Actually, my purpose in telling you about these statistics is not to alarm you, but to inform you. We can try to ignore the obvious when it comes to our daughters' sexuality, but it doesn't change the cold, hard facts. Each one of those young girls out there experimenting with sex must be someone's daughter. Is she yours?

Perhaps not. After all, even if more than 60% of twelfth-grade girls have engaged in sexual intercourse, that still means that almost 40% have not. Perhaps your daughter is in the latter group. But are you really willing to gamble on your daughter's health, and on the risk that she could become pregnant, simply because you feel uncomfortable talking to her about safe sex?

Sexually transmitted disease (STD)

Also known as sexually transmitted infection (STI), or venereal disease (VD), this category includes any infection that can be transmitted from one person to another through any sexual contact, including oral sex.

I thought not. So let's start by discussing **sexually transmitted diseases (STDs)**.

The first thing I want to emphasize is that all it takes to expose a young woman to any STD is one partner. That's all—one partner. And all it takes to expose a young woman to any STD is one sexual episode. That's all—one episode. Although the incidence of STDs rises with the number of partners a young woman has had, as a gynecologist I have seen many distraught females who have had sex with their first sexual partner for the first time and they have contracted one, two, or even three infections. And in many instances the girl's partner never even knew he had a disease.

How is it possible that the guy didn't know? Because—drum roll, please—many STDs cause little or no obvious signs in men. That's right. Men can be clueless that they're infectious. And just to compound the unfairness, I'm sure you and your daughter will be interested to know that even when a guy does discover that he has an STD, he typically can easily receive treatment without any of the lifelong health consequences that afflict females. (Yes, when it comes to males and females, life is unfair—but we already knew that because of pantyhose.)

39. How important are condoms in preventing STDs?

Because of these facts, I constantly emphasize to my young patients the need to protect themselves. And the best form of protection, besides abstinence, is a low-tech **condom**. Because **semen** is often the source of transmission when it comes to sexually transmitted diseases, if a girl doesn't expose herself to it, she is going to be much, much safer.

"Use a condom. . . . Use a condom. . . . Use a condom. . . ." That refrain should play over and over in every female's mind when she engages in behavior that may subject her to even the slightest risk of contracting a sexually transmitted disease. Notions such as "Just this once . . .," or "But he seems really nice . . .," or "I'm too drunk to care . . .," should NEVER be allowed to trump the "Use a condom" mantra.

When it comes to condom use (which I'll discuss in more detail in the chapter about birth control), your daughter

Condom

A thin sheath, often made of latex, which is placed over the penis to capture semen for the purpose of preventing pregnancy and the transmission of infection.

Semen

The fluid containing sperm that is released from the penis during ejaculation. This fluid helps the sperm reach the egg for fertilization.

should realize a couple of things at the outset. First, yes, it may be a little awkward to stop in the "middle of the action" and ask whether a partner has "protection." But if there is so little communication and connection between the two of them that this simple, understandable question is unbearably awkward, then she shouldn't be physically intimate with him in the first place.

And second, your daughter should know that wearing a condom during sexual activity isn't quite as much fun for the guy. No matter the type of condom or its thinness, and no matter what some advocates may try to claim, its use somewhat reduces the sensation that a partner feels on his penis. That's why she needs to be prepared for the fact that some guys will try to convince a girl—sometimes repeatedly and persistently—that he shouldn't have to wear one.

Your daughter shouldn't fall for any reason her partner may try to give her about why he shouldn't have to use a condom. If a little, fleeting, extra sensation is worth more to the guy than your daughter's long-tem health, then she shouldn't care about his pleasure at all. Moreover, a guy is going to get *plenty* of satisfaction out of the deal anyway, no matter what. Therefore, affording your daughter this dramatically increased protection just makes sense. So, to recap, the proper refrain always is, "Use a condom. . . . Use a condom. . . . Use a condom. . . ."

40. How common are STD infections?

You may be saying to yourself, "You know what? I really don't think STDs are a problem with the types of kids my daughter hangs out with." Maybe you're right. But keep this statistic in mind—the Centers for Disease Control and Prevention released a study in

March of 2008 that shows that more than one in four adolescent females in the United States has a sexually transmitted infection (STI). That's right. Twenty-six percent of American girls between the ages of 14 and 19 have the human papillomavirus (HPV), chlamydia, herpes simplex virus type 2 (HSV-2), and/or trichomoniasis. Even among the girls reporting only one lifetime sexual partner, 20% had at least one STD.

The question you probably have in your mind right now is, "Why is the rate of infection so high for adolescent girls?" Well, there are a number of reasons for it. First, the adolescent **cervix** is particularly vulnerable to infections such as HPV, chlamydia, and gonorrhea because it is still developing. Second, the number of antibodies that fight infection isn't as high in male and female adolescents as it is in older adults. And third, adolescents may be more prone to engage in high-risk sexual behavior.

This high-risk behavior may be caused by several factors. For instance, those "raging hormones" we hear so much about really do exist. (Remember?) Unfortunately, the power they exert can sometimes override a girl's common sense about protecting herself. Further, adolescents often have a certain sense of invincibility. They believe that bad things are remote in possibility and happen to someone else rather than to themselves. Or, a girl might be engaging in risky behavior because of peer pressure or manipulation and control by her partner. And finally, don't overlook the effects of drugs and alcohol on the types of sexual behavior that an adolescent girl will engage in. (Did you know that 28% of all adolescents report that they used alcohol *before they turned 13*?)

The adolescent cervix is particularly vulnerable to infections such as HPV, chlamydia, and gonorrhea because it is still developing.

Cervix

The organ at the lower end of the uterus that separates the uterus from the vagina. The cervix plays an important role in holding a developing fetus inside the uterus until labor begins. In addition, the cervix is the site from which samples are obtained for Pap smear testing, and it can be the site of abnormal growths such as cancer.

There are almost too many different types of STDs to mention in this book. However, it is worthwhile to cover the signs, symptoms, and treatments of the most common infections.

Human papillomavirus is one of the most common and potentially harmful sexually transmitted diseases. Although researchers have now developed vaccines that can greatly reduce the threat of this virus to young women, there has been some controversy about this important issue. As a result, I've decided to cover this topic in depth in a separate chapter. By analyzing the information contained there, you can make an educated and informed decision about whether your daughter should receive the HPV vaccine.

41. What is chlamydia?

Chlamydia is one of the four most common sexually transmitted diseases. It is caused by bacteria, and in 2006, more than one million cases of chlamydia were reported in the United States.

As many as 25% of all males who have chlamydia have no symptoms. Those who do have symptoms experience a burning sensation while urinating, discharge from the penis or rectum, testicular pain, and rectal pain.

Unlike a number of other STDs, a relatively low percentage of women (only about one-third) who have chlamydia experience symptoms.

Interestingly, unlike a number of other STDs, a relatively low percentage of women (only about one-third) who have chlamydia experience symptoms. That's why the Centers for Disease Control and Prevention and the American College of Obstetricians and Gynecologists recommend yearly screening of all sexually active adolescent and young adult females up to 25 years of age (and older if they have new partners). Those women who do have symptoms from chlamydia experience burning while urinating, vaginal discharge, painful intercourse, and rectal pain.

If a woman's chlamydia infection remains untreated, it can lead to pelvic inflammatory disease, infection of the **fallopian tubes,** and ultimately, **infertility**. Scarring of the fallopian tubes from a chlamydia infection also increases the risk of a tubal pregnancy, which can be hazardous to the health of the mother. Further, a chlamydia infection can cause a woman to deliver prematurely, and it can be passed on to a newborn in the form of an eye infection or pneumonia.

If a woman contracts chlamydia, the treatment is quite simple. It merely consists of taking one of several common antibiotics. Both partners must be treated before they can resume intercourse.

There is no immunity gained from a chlamydia infection. That means that a woman can get repeated infections with repeated exposure. Chlamydia is found in cervical secretions and semen, so condoms provide significant protection to both partners.

42. What is gonorrhea?

Gonorrhea is a common STD that is caused by bacteria that thrive in the female and male genital tracts. It is spread through contact with the penis, vagina, mouth, and **anus**. Ejaculation by the male partner doesn't have to occur for transmission to take place.

Approximately 700,000 new cases of gonorrhea occur each year, and the biggest group affected is sexually active teenagers. Although some men have no symptoms when they get gonorrhea, other men experience burning while urinating, penile discharge, and tender testicles.

Fallopian tubes

Two long, tubular structures that are attached to the top sides of the uterus. Fertilization of the egg takes place in the fallopian tubes. Each fallopian tube lies in close proximity to each ovary.

Infertility

The inability to get pregnant without assistance.

Anus

The opening of the rectum to the outside of the body.

Pelvic abscess

A localized area of pus in the pelvic region.

Chronic pelvic pain

Persistent pelvic pain that is not alleviated by usual means. Certain disorders such as endometriosis, fibroids, cysts, and pelvic adhesions can often be the cause of chronic pelvic pain, but in many cases, no cause is found.

Ectopic pregnancy

A pregnancy that occurs outside of the uterine cavity. Sites can include fallopian tubes, ovaries, the cervix, and the abdomen.

The best protection from gonorrhea, other than abstinence or being in a long-term mutually monogamous relationship, is a latex condom.

Monogamous

Being in a relationship between two people with no other partners.

Oral sex

A sexual act involving oral stimulation of the genital area.

Women who contract gonorrhea typically notice a vaginal discharge, a burning sensation while urinating, or irregular bleeding. However, these symptoms may not appear until the infection has spread considerably. Both sexes also may experience anal pain.

Gonorrhea is a common cause of pelvic inflammatory disease, an infection in the upper genital region that can cause a woman to become infertile. Gonorrhea can cause fallopian tube damage and **pelvic abscesses**, which, in turn, can lead to **chronic pelvic pain** and an increased risk of an **ectopic pregnancy**.

Screening for gonorrhea is recommended for all sexually active females until the age of 25, and for any woman older than that who has a new sexual partner. This can be done with a simple test in the doctor's office. Moreover, gonorrhea usually can be easily treated with a course of antibiotics. (However, there has been an increasing problem with antibiotic-resistant strains of gonorrhea.) The best protection from gonorrhea, other than abstinence or being in a long-term mutually **monogamous** relationship, is a latex condom.

43. What is genital herpes?

Genital herpes is caused by the herpes simplex virus, type 1 and type 2. The herpes simplex type 1 virus is a very common infection; it is usually found in the mouth and is the cause of the cold sores and fever blisters you see on people's lips.

Most of the genital herpes infections are caused by the herpes simplex type 2 virus. It is found in the genital region. Interestingly, recent reports show an increase in type 1 herpes on the genital region in women who have **oral sex** performed on them by an infected partner.

With the first outbreak, a herpes infection typically results in painful blisters that later become painful sores that may last for weeks. Later outbreaks are usually not as severe and typically decrease in frequency over time.

Genital herpes is very common. It affects approximately 45 million Americans aged 12 or older. It's possible for an infected person who has no symptoms to transmit an infection to a partner because the skin in the infected region can still shed the virus. While normally not dangerous in a person with a normal immune system, genital herpes can cause physical pain and, of course, significant psychological distress. An infection is life-long. There is no cure. However there are medications that can help suppress outbreaks, diminish the symptoms, and reduce transmission to partners.

To reduce the risk of infection, latex condoms are a must. Further, it's important not to have any type of sexual contact during an outbreak. And finally, your daughter should be aware that there is a small risk of pregnant women transmitting the herpes virus to their babies during labor.

44. What is HIV?

HIV stands for human immunodeficiency virus, and it is the virus that causes AIDS. Although I have seen extremely little of this infection in my practice, the test for it is the most requested—and most feared—among my patients coming in for STD screening.

In 2006, the Centers for Disease Control and Prevention estimated that there were 56,300 new cases of HIV in the United States. In 2004, the most recent year that statistics of this nature are readily available, 13% of all new HIV cases occurred among adolescents and young adults 13 to 24 years of age. Moreover, women of all ages now comprise approximately one quarter of all new HIV cases in America. It's important to note that with vaginal intercourse, a woman has a greater chance than the man of contracting HIV.

HIV does its dirty work by attacking the immune system and weakening it, thereby making it far more susceptible to uncommon life-threatening infections. Latex condoms, if used consistently and properly, provide significant protection. Transmission is increased if there are open sores from herpes or syphilis.

When an HIV-positive person is infected with an uncommon infection, they are said to have contracted Acquired Immune Deficiency Syndrome (AIDS). If untreated, AIDS is fatal. However, although there is no cure, there are successful drug suppression treatments that decrease the number of AIDS cases in HIV-positive people.

45. What is syphilis?

There were 36,000 cases of syphilis reported in 2006, and almost 10,000 of these were new cases. Although there was a decrease in the number of cases reported in the 1990s, there has been a troubling increase recently. Syphilis infections are most common in women between the ages of 20 and 24. The syphilis bacteria are transmitted from open sores that can be anywhere on the male or female genital area.

There are different stages of a syphilis infection. The primary stage, when the open sore is present, is easily treated with an antibiotic. Unfortunately, however, many people don't seek treatment promptly because the sores are not painful. Those who go untreated progress to the secondary stage of syphilis, which results in a rash, often on the feet and hands, along with symptoms of swollen lymph nodes, fever, headache, and fatigue. These symptoms can be vague and often go undiagnosed. A continued untreated infection can progress years later to the late stage of syphilis. This is the stage where syphilis can infect the brain and internal organs and cause dementia, blindness, and even death. The second and late stages are treated with long courses of antibiotics.

Syphilis is usually diagnosed with a blood test. Pregnant women can pass a syphilis infection onto their babies with serious consequences for the child, and that's why all pregnant women are screened for syphilis during their pregnancies. The simple use of a condom will help prevent the transmission of this ugly disease.

46. What is hepatitis B?

Hepatitis is a general term that doctors use to describe inflammation of the liver. One common cause of hepatitis is the hepatitis B virus. Infection with this virus typically occurs when a person comes in contact with infected blood, semen, or other body fluids, or is exposed to dirty needles and injectable drug equipment previously used by an infected person.

In 2006, 46,000 new cases of hepatitis B were reported. A person infected with this virus may have symptoms of **jaundice** (which is yellowing of the skin), or may have no symptoms at all. Some people will clear their hepatitis B infection on their own and be completely cured. In other cases, people will suffer from a chronic or long-term infection that can result in liver damage, liver failure, and even death.

Jaundice
A yellowing of the skin and eyes often caused by liver disease.

There are approximately 1.25 million people who suffer from a chronic hepatitis B infection. There is no cure for it, but there are treatments that may delay damage to the liver. The hepatitis B vaccine is one of the vaccines that all babies receive shortly after birth to prevent newborns from getting an infection. In fact, this vaccine is available to all people who may be at risk of a hepatitis B infection.

47. What is hepatitis C?

The hepatitis C virus is the most common cause of hepatitis.

The hepatitis C virus is the most common cause of hepatitis. In 2006, 3.2 million Americans were reported to have a chronic hepatitis C infection.

Transmission of this virus occurs through contact with infected blood, infected body fluids, or infected needles and other injectable drug equipment. Although hepatitis C has been reported in women who have no other risk factors than sexual contact with an infected person, studies done on partners of hepatitis C infected people show only a 1.5% transmission rate. Nonetheless, the risk of contracting hepatitis C is one more reason why your daughter should insist that her partner wears a condom.

The symptoms of a hepatitis C viral infection initially range from a mild illness to no symptoms at all. However, many initial infections proceed on to chronic infections that cause liver failure and death. There is no vaccine; however, there have been some promising treatments that may clear the virus from the system.

48. What is trichomoniasis?

Trichomoniasis is an STD that is caused by an invisible parasite that lives in the vagina and male urethra.

More than 7 million Americans are infected with this disease annually.

Women who contract trichomoniasis typically have a frothy green-yellow vaginal discharge. They also often experience itching, burning, or bleeding after intercourse. Men may have no symptoms.

Trichomoniasis is transmitted through male-female intercourse or vulva-to-vulva (the skin area outside the vagina) contact. It is easily treated with a course of medicine, and in order to avoid reinfection, both partners should be treated and retested negative before any further sexual contact.

49. What is molluscum contagiosum?

I know you've probably never heard of this disease, but it's a skin infection caused by a common virus called a DNA poxvirus. Younger children can get it through common towel use, the shared use of athletic equipment, and non-sexual skin-to-skin contact. Older children and adults can get it from all these sources, *plus* sexual contact.

Molluscum contagiosum causes small, firm bumps on the skin with a central "belly button" appearance. The bumps can number into the hundreds and may cause itching and pain. In children they are present on the trunk and extremities. When this infection appears in young adults, it is often on the genital and inner thigh region and is considered an STD.

This is not a life-threatening infection, but it's often hard to get rid of due to its contagious nature. A trip to the doctor's office is required for treatment and usually involves freezing or physical eradication of the bumps.

I see this infection periodically in my office, and repeat visits are often needed to get rid of it completely. Regular washing and limitation of sexual partners are measures that can be taken to try to reduce the chance of this infection.

PART SEVEN

The Human Papillomavirus Vaccine

What cancers are associated with HPV?

How is HPV transmitted?

What protection do the HPV vaccines provide?

More . . .

Human Papillomavirus (HPV) is the most common sexually transmitted disease in the United States. In fact, researchers estimate that 80% of all women will have acquired an HPV infection by the time they reach age 50. That statistic is astounding.

Thankfully, most of the women who become infected with HPV will clear the virus (which means that their bodies will manage to defeat it and there will be no signs of it remaining in a woman's system), and they will have no lasting effects from it. However, those women who don't clear the virus have an increased risk of getting, among other ailments, vulvar, vaginal, anal, and cervical cancer, as well as genital warts.

50. What are genital warts?

Genital warts

Warty structures on the genital region caused by the human papillomavirus. These are considered a sexually transmitted infection. Topical medications or surgical removal are used to treat them.

Interestingly, the prospect of getting **genital warts** seems to upset some women just as much as the chance of getting cancer. (The more precise term is "anogenital" warts because the anal region can be involved too. Anal cancer is on the rise due to anal HPV.)

One million new cases of anogenital warts are diagnosed each year. The majority of these cases last more than four months and require repeated trips to the doctor for treatment. These treatments can include such steps as applying a topical substance to the lesions, or freezing or lasering them off. Furthermore, recurrence of the disease is common, resulting in an additional series of trips to the doctor. (If you explain this process to your daughter in painstaking detail, it may prove to be a powerful motivator for her to ensure that *all* of her sex partners wear condoms *all* of the time.)

Certain types of HPV are associated with cancers of the cervix, vagina, anus, and vulva.

51. What cancers are associated with HPV?

Unfortunately, as I noted earlier, certain types of HPV are associated with cancers of the cervix, vagina, anus, and vulva. In fact, in 2007, more than 11,000 new cases of cervical cancer were diagnosed in this country, and almost 4,000 women died from it. This number would have been much higher if Pap testing wasn't such a standard practice in this country.

Tragically, Pap testing is not a routine procedure worldwide, particularly in developing countries where medical care is scarce or completely unattainable. As a result, each year more than a half-million women around the globe develop cervical cancer, and a quarter-million women die from it. In fact, cervical cancer is the second-leading cause of cancer deaths for women worldwide.

52. How is HPV transmitted?

The human papillomavirus is transmitted through direct skin-to-skin contact, usually during vaginal or anal intercourse. The majority of these infections occur during the first few years of sexual activity. Although the risk of getting HPV is directly related to the number of partners a female has, it's also important to note that even if a girl or a woman has only one sex partner, and that one sex partner has HPV, she can get infected. It's also important to note that the adolescent cervix seems especially vulnerable to the HPV virus. This may help to explain why the number of infections seems peculiarly high in the early years of sexual activity.

Although the majority of HPV infections are cleared from a woman's body spontaneously, a certain percentage of HPV infections are particularly persistent. Moreover, there are other factors that can place a female at increased risk for a persistent HPV infection. Specifically, if a woman smokes, is over age 30, is infected with multiple HPV subtypes, has a suppressed

The Human Papillomavirus Vaccine

immune system, or is using oral contraceptives, an HPV infection can be harder to clear.

53. What are the HPV vaccines?

Because of the seriousness of this problem, scientists spent a lot of time researching HPV. Finally, in 2006, the Food and Drug Administration (FDA) approved a much-anticipated HPV vaccine called Gardasil. This enormously important vaccine protects against four types of HPV—two that cause 90% of anogenital warts, and two that cause 70% of cervical cancers. It is important to note that there are more than 40 subtypes of genital HPV, so not all types are covered by the Gardasil vaccine. Gardasil is approved for both females and males from the ages of 9 through 26 years.

Another HPV vaccine was approved by the FDA in November 2009. This vaccine is called Cervarix and is approved for use in females aged 10 through 25 years. Cervarix is designed to protect against two types of HPV that cause cervical cancer. Both Gardasil and Cervarix consist of *non*infectious, virus-*like* particles. In other words, you can't get HPV from receiving these vaccines. Gardasil and Cervarix are given by a series of three injections. The second shot is typically given 1 or 2 months after the first one, and the final shot is typically given 6 months after the first one. Past medical studies of Gardasil have demonstrated that it provides protection for 5 years. Ongoing studies are being conducted to determine if it actually provides protection for at least 14 years. Cervarix has been found to provide protection for 6 years.

*Both Gardasil and Cervarix consist of non*infectious, *virus-*like *particles. In other words, you can't get HPV from receiving these vaccines.*

54. What protection do the HPV vaccines provide?

Large scientific studies (one of them included more than 20,000 women between the ages of 16 and 26) have shown that women who were not previously exposed to HPV, and who completed the three-injection series of Gardasil, received virtually complete protection against the four types of HPV covered by the vaccine. Specifically, Gardasil provided protection against 99% of HPV 16-related lesions, 100% of HPV 18-related lesions, 99% of anogenital warts, and 100% of **precancerous** HPV 16- and 18-related vaginal and vulvar lesions.

Even in the patients who failed to complete the three-injection series or who were HPV-positive prior to the vaccine, there still was a sizeable reduction in HPV 16- and 18-related precancerous lesions. (It was a 42% and 81% decrease, respectively.) Moreover, it also has been recently discovered that Gardasil seems to provide cross-protection against other types of HPV that are not included in the vaccine. This positive development is the result of the similarity of proteins among the various types of HPV. Researchers are hopeful that this signals added protection for women against genital cancers.

Cervarix also provides protection against the two more common high-risk HPV types, HPV 16 and 18. The primary clinical study for Cervarix showed it was 93% effective in preventing precancerous cervical lesions caused by HPV 16 and 18 in females who had no prior known exposure to these HPV types.

55. Are the HPV vaccines recommended for adolescent girls?

The Advisory Committee on Immunization Practices (which consists of 15 experts on vaccine-preventable diseases who advise the Secretary of Health and Human Services and the CDC) recommends that the HPV vaccine should be administered to 11- and 12-year-old

Precancerous

A condition in which there is the potential that a cancer will form. Precancerous cells on the cervix, if left untreated, may have the ability to form cervical cancer.

girls as part of a routine vaccination schedule. The American College of Obstetricians and Gynecologists, the Society for Adolescent Medicine, and the American Academy of Family Physicians have made similar recommendations.

When the HPV vaccination recommendations were first announced, there understandably was a lot of pushback from parents who initially felt that it was unnecessary to vaccinate their preteen-aged daughters against a sexually transmitted infection. However, as the word has gotten out that the whole point of the program is to inoculate children *before* they are exposed to HPV, the resistance has waned. Nevertheless, whenever it comes to vaccines—or any other type of medication or medical treatment—it is wise to become fully informed about them.

56. What are the side effects of the HPV vaccines?

For almost all patients, the HPV vaccines are well-tolerated. Common side effects include pain, swelling, and redness at the injection site. These side effects were rated as mild to moderate by the majority of participants. However, if a patient is known to be hypersensitive to the active or inactive substances in the vaccine, she shouldn't receive it. Similarly, if a patient develops a hypersensitivity or allergic reaction after one injection, then the remaining injections obviously should be withheld. The HPV vaccines have not been approved for use in pregnant women, and their safety while a woman is breastfeeding is unknown. Because light-headedness or fainting can be a reaction of receiving any shot, a 15-minute wait time at the doctor's office is recommended after receiving Gardasil or Cervarix.

In the summer of 2008, news stories surfaced regarding reports of serious adverse events associated with Gardasil. However, the CDC and the FDA examined these reports, and after careful analysis, concluded that young girls still should be vaccinated. Specifically, the CDC and the FDA made the following findings.

A total of 9,749 adverse events were reported from the start of Gardasil vaccinations in June 2006 through June 2008. Approximately 94% of these adverse events were classified as non-serious. They included such complaints as injection-site pain, headaches, nausea, fever, and fainting.

The remaining 6% of the adverse events were deemed to be serious. In fact, 20 deaths reportedly occurred at some point after a girl received this HPV vaccine. This number obviously sounds *very* alarming. However, the CDC and the FDA analyzed these cases closely and ultimately determined that there appeared to be no common link among the causes of death in these girls and, therefore, they concluded that there wasn't anything to indicate that the vaccine was really the cause. In fact, when autopsy results were available, the cause of these deaths was shown to be unrelated to the vaccine. Keep in mind that 24 million doses of Gardasil have been given as of May 2009.

Other serious adverse events investigated by the CDC and the FDA included blood clot disorders, but most of these cases occurred in females with risk factors for clotting. There also were cases of Guillain-Barré Syndrome (GBS), a rare neurological disorder that is seen most frequently in adolescents. However, the CDC and the FDA found no increase in GBS cases beyond

The Human Papillomavirus Vaccine

the number typically expected among girls who received Gardasil. It is reassuring to know that there are three vaccine safety monitoring systems that continuously collect data on all vaccines to watch for any adverse effects.

And finally, if you've been following the debate about other vaccines, you'll be happy to know that Gardasil and Cervarix contain no thimerosal.

57. Will insurance pay for the HPV vaccines?

Gardasil typically is covered by insurance plans. For the uninsured, the Vaccines for Children Program (which is federally funded) provides the vaccine to children who are covered by Medicaid or who are Medicaid-eligible, as well as to the uninsured, American Indians/Native Americans, and Alaskan natives. While there is no federally funded program to cover the cost of Gardasil for uninsured adults, the manufacturer of Gardasil has established a vaccination assistance program for uninsured women whose income is below 200% of the poverty level and for others on an individual case-by-case basis. It is anticipated that Cervarix will be covered by insurance plans as well.

58. What exactly does an HPV infection mean to my daughter?

When my patients come in with questions about vaccinating their daughters, I try to enlighten them about the far reaching effects of HPV. I've already covered the health consequences that can result from becoming infected with HPV such as genital warts and cancer, but there even are adverse consequences that can stem from the testing and treatment of women who have HPV.

Nowadays, doctors are careful not to overtreat a young woman's cervix. However, because HPV can be persistent, oftentimes it is necessary to perform a colposcopy on a patient. A **colposcopy** is an uncomfortable, longer-than-usual pelvic exam involving a careful look at the cervix that is accompanied by the performance of small biopsies. Often no further treatment is necessary other than more frequent Pap smears, but this testing requires additional visits to the doctor's office.

At other times, treatment for HPV is required, and this consists of freezing, or even removing a small portion of, the cervix. Most of the time this completes treatment and the patient is simply followed with periodic Pap smears. However, women who have had these procedures performed on them need to be followed more closely during pregnancy. Occasionally, bed rest, frequent sonograms, and even a stitch in the cervix are required to support the growing pregnancy. While most women complete their pregnancies without a problem, there is a higher incidence of preterm delivery in these types of patients.

But that's not all. Sometimes the abnormal cells caused by HPV return as patients grow older. In fact, some women decide to have hysterectomies after child bearing due to the persistence of Pap abnormalities and the presence of high-risk HPV so as to rid themselves of the risk of cervical cancer.

59. Should my daughter receive the HPV vaccine?

Above, I have listed the primary factors you need to weigh when making the important decision about whether your daughter should receive the HPV vaccine. You shouldn't make this decision lightly, you should do so in consultation with your own doctor, and you should be mindful of the fact that additional information

> **Colposcopy**
>
> An office procedure in which the cervix is viewed through a colposcope, or magnifying instrument. A colposcopy is the test done to further evaluate the cervix after an abnormal Pap smear. Often small biopsies are performed during this procedure.

could come to light in the future that could alter the equation.

But having said that, I hope you will be guided by the facts and the science related to this matter rather than by emotions, rumors, unfounded suppositions, and inertia. I don't want to paint too stark a picture, but as a physician, this is how I see it: On one side of the equation you have the downsides of the HPV vaccine—if your daughter receives it, she may experience temporary injection-site pain, headache, nausea, fever, and fainting. On the other side of the equation, however, is this simple fact—if your daughter does *not* receive the vaccine, she is highly likely to contract the human papillomavirus. If she does, your daughter is at increased risk for genital warts, cervical cancer, vulvar cancer, vaginal cancer, and anal cancer; she may be subjected to unpleasant examination procedures and treatments to address her HPV infection; and she may experience complications during pregnancy.

Now you must decide what's best for *your* daughter.

PART EIGHT

Birth Control

What are the benefits of abstinence?

What are barrier methods of contraception?

What does my daughter need to know about birth control pills?

More . . .

When a mother starts thinking about having a conversation with her daughter about sex and birth control, she often worries about how best to handle it. After all, before the mom can even focus on the substance of the discussion, she has to focus on the timing. Some moms fear that if they have "the talk" too soon, their daughters will view it as a green light to begin experimenting with sex at an early age. (This is the "It will put ideas in her head!" argument.) Other moms fear that if they have "the talk" too late, their daughters will end up having unprotected sex because they didn't know any better. (This is the "You're WHAT!?!?! Just wait until your father gets home!" argument.)

The truth of the matter is that kids typically know the basics of sex at a pretty young age. Most public schools do a good job of teaching sex education classes, often when the kids are in fifth grade. When you learn that this block of instruction is being covered in school, you should go out of your way to ensure that you can spend some private, quiet time with your daughter so that she can spontaneously raise with you any questions she might have about the topic. If she doesn't initiate the conversation, you should.

Needless to say, you should answer your daughter's questions fully, openly, and honestly. And remember— you can make your daughter feel comfortable talking with you about sex if you consistently demonstrate that you feel comfortable talking with her about sex. Keep in mind, also, that when it comes to sex, the phrase "the talk" is very misleading. In actuality, starting when she's young, you will need to engage in a series of mini-talks with your daughter about this crucial subject.

During these conversations, it's very important for you to share with your daughter your views and your values regarding sexual activity. Some moms steer clear of this part of the conversation because they don't want to be seen as being uncool or judgmental. But taking such a position is, in reality, an abdication of a mother's parental responsibility. Talking to your daughter about being safe, about being responsible, about making choices that are right for her, about maintaining her self-respect, and about being true to her beliefs is far from being old-fashioned.

60. Is my daughter too young for birth control?

So, when do you have to start worrying about birth control for your daughter? Well, every girl is different, and it's critical to remember that point. Nevertheless, it's oftentimes helpful to look at broad-based scientific studies to get a sense of what's happening in this modern age of adolescent sex.

One such study is the Youth Risk Behavior Survey (YRBS) that has been conducted bi-annually since 1990 by the CDC. This study consists of school-based surveys of students in grades 9 through 12. In 2007, the YRBS showed that 47.8% of all high school students nationwide reported that they had engaged in sexual intercourse. Specifically, approximately 27% of 9th grade females, 42% of 10th grade females, 54% of 11th grade females, and 66% of 12th grade females said they had had sexual intercourse.

The YRBS also reveals other interesting statistics. For instance, 20% of 12th grade females reported having four or more sexual partners. Additionally, only 62% of the students who reported being sexually active said that during their last incident of sexual intercourse, either they or their partner had used a condom. Only an additional 16% of all currently sexually active students said that either they or their partner had used birth control pills during their last sexual encounter. (Now you know why it's called the Youth *Risk* Behavior Survey.)

These statistics show why it's so important for us to stress to our daughters the need for birth control if they become sexually active, and for us to begin doing so while our daughters are still young. Therefore, let's turn our attention to the various types of birth control, their proper use, and their rate of effectiveness.

Kama says:

Studies have shown that human contact is a basic human need. Yet many parents are so overwhelmed with lives that are jammed packed from sun-up until bedtime, that sadly, many children are deprived of this. A hug, a kiss, a pat on the back reinforces a child's sense of security and feelings of self-worth. Simply put, if children are deprived of nurturing physical contact, they may be more apt to seek an inappropriate avenue to fill that need.

61. What are the benefits of abstinence?

The very first thing that everyone needs to think about and acknowledge is the fact that, even in the twenty-first century, **abstinence** is the "gold standard" when it comes to contraception. Simply stated, if your daughter doesn't engage in sexual activity of any kind, she won't get pregnant and she won't be exposing herself to sexually transmitted diseases. No one can make that claim for any other type of contraception method. Period.

Abstinence

The act of not partici-pating in sexual activity.

Now, some people will claim that advocating abstinence is unrealistic and naïve. That's certainly true when we're talking about the population as a whole. The plain truth is that a lot of young people are going to have sex regardless of their parents' wishes and actions. But abstinence can be the right choice for any particular individual. We do our daughters a grave disservice if we don't discuss with them our morals and our values when it comes to sexual activity, and part of that discussion needs to be about the unique benefits of abstinence.

If, however, your daughter chooses to engage in sexual intercourse, she should be fully aware of her options when it comes to birth control. There are a lot of choices out there. In fact, the various forms of birth control can be grouped into seven categories. These are: rhythm, withdrawal, barrier, hormonal, emergency, intrauterine devices, and permanent. Let's go through them one at a time.

62. What is the rhythm method?

In order to be able to successfully use this method, a woman needs to be familiar with the length of her menstrual cycle, and she needs to be able to notice changes indicating **ovulation**. Specifically, with the rhythm method a woman has to track her **basal body temperature** and engage in **cervical mucus** monitoring to figure out when she's **fertile**. Then she has to make sure that she doesn't have intercourse during the time that the **egg** is present so that she can avoid becoming pregnant.

Because of the imprecision and difficulties inherent to such an approach, it's been reported that the failure of the rhythm method can be as high as 25%.

I certainly don't recommend the rhythm method to my young patients. They're typically not willing to put in the effort to monitor their body changes, their menstrual cycles often are not as regular as older women's,

Ovulation
The release of the egg from the ovary that occurs monthly. The egg is then picked up by the fallopian tube and awaits fertilization.

Basal body temperature
The early morning temperature of the human body.

Cervical mucus
The mucus in the cervical canal that is produced by cervical glands and provides protection against pelvic infections and pregnancy. Cervical mucus changes temporarily during ovulation to enhance the chance of pregnancy.

Fertile
The ability to get pregnant without difficulty.

Egg
Found in the ovary, the egg is a microscopic cell that is released from the ovary at the time of ovulation. The egg contains the woman's genetic material and combines with the sperm to form the embryo.

Birth Control

and too often their sexual desires overpower what their bodies are telling them about their fertility.

63. What is coitus interruptus?

Coitus interruptus is also known as the "withdrawal method." This method of birth control has been around for thousands of years and is still used today by millions and millions of couples worldwide.

The effectiveness of this method is dependent upon whether the male maintains sufficient control that he can completely pull his penis out of his partner's vagina (and away from her vulva) before he ejaculates. However, even if he can, there still remains one small problem—**sperm**. These "little fellas" sometimes decide to hitch a ride in the man's *pre*-ejaculate fluid, and then are deposited in the woman's vagina, thus potentially fertilizing her egg.

The perfect use failure rate for the withdrawal method is estimated at 4%. However, researchers have found that the *typical* failure rate can be as much as 27%.

64. What are barrier methods of contraception?

Barrier methods work by preventing the man's sperm from reaching the woman's egg. There are several types, including spermicide, condoms, cervical caps, diaphragms, and the sponge.

Spermicides are chemical barriers that come in the form of vaginal creams, gels, foams, films, and suppositories. They work by being applied in a woman's vagina where they can then kill or inactivate sperm that are deposited by the man. Among other benefits, spermicides are inexpensive and are readily available over the counter.

Sperm

The cells in the semen that fertilize the female egg. Sperm contain the father's genetic material.

It's important for a woman to read the directions of the particular type of spermicide that she decides upon. Some need to be inserted into the vagina just prior to the act of intercourse, while others require insertion 10 to 30 minutes before intercourse so that they have time to dissolve in the vagina and become activated. (This usually holds true for the film and tablet forms of spermicides.)

You may recall that manufacturers used to advertise the supposed protective effect of Nonoxynol 9 (N9), a chemical found in many spermicides. Specifically, it was claimed that N9 would protect against the transmission of HIV and other STDs. However, in 2003, the FDA warned the public that the results of a large study showed that N9 did *not* protect women from these diseases. In fact, it was disclosed that the use of N9 products could cause vaginal and rectal irritation, which, in turn, could actually *increase* the risk of contracting HIV and other STDs. In 2007, the FDA finally required all products that contain N9 to carry a warning about these risks. Accordingly, I think it would be wise to steer clear of these products.

65. How do condoms protect against STDs and pregnancy?

Condoms, of course, are thin sheaths that are placed over a man's penis in order to capture the sperm-filled semen and thereby prevent it from fertilizing the woman's egg.

There's a difference between semen and sperm. Semen is the fluid that a man ejaculates as he reaches orgasm. Sperm are the little swimmers *within* the semen that actually swim up the woman's fallopian tubes and fertilize the egg.

Condoms are usually made of latex, and they are inexpensive and easy to obtain over the counter. (Non-latex condoms are made of animal tissue and provide less protection against STDs than the latex ones. Accordingly, you and your daughter should avoid them.) Latex condoms should be used only with water-based lubricants because oil-based lubricants such as creams, vegetable oils, and petroleum jelly can damage them.

Latex condoms should be used only with water-based lubricants because oil-based lubricants such as creams, vegetable oils, and petroleum jelly can damage them.

To use it correctly, the man should take a new, rolled-up condom, place it over the end of his erect penis, hold the tip of the condom to allow some extra space for the semen to go when he ejaculates, and then unroll the rest of the condom down over the shaft of his penis. Right after he ejaculates, the man should grasp the condom at the base of his shaft and then withdraw his penis from the woman's vagina. This procedure prevents the man's semen from spilling into the woman's vagina once he becomes flaccid after ejaculation.

Condoms should be used only one time. They provide important protection against many STDs, but many people, both women *and* men, are surprised to find that the failure rate of condoms is approximately 15%.

66. What is a female condom?

A female condom may sound like an oxymoron to some people, but it's not. It consists of a plastic pouch that has a closed inner ring that is placed in the vagina next to the cervix. The open, outer ring then extends past the vaginal opening. Any lubricant can be used with a female condom and it, too, is available over the counter.

When using a female condom, after the man ejaculates, the woman should squeeze and twist the outer rings of the pouch to close it. She then should pull the entire condom out of her vagina and discard it. Because, among other issues, semen sometimes spills out of the female condom when the woman is trying to twist it closed, the failure rate is an unimpressive 21%.

67. How does a diaphragm work?

A diaphragm is a rubber dome that fits in the vagina and covers the cervix. It is both a physical and chemical barrier method. A woman who wishes to use a diaphragm as her method of birth control needs to visit a doctor to be fitted for the correct size and to receive a prescription for the diaphragm.

Diaphragms must be inserted prior to intercourse and then left in place for at least 6 hours after intercourse. Their effectiveness is dependent on the woman also using a spermicidal jelly at the same time as the diaphragm. Only water-based lubricants should be used with the diaphragm because oil-based lubricants can cause deterioration of the rubber.

There is an increased risk for bladder infections with the use of a diaphragm. Further, typical failure rates hover around 16%. In my experience as a gynecologist, teenagers don't use this method very much.

68. Are cervical caps similar to diaphragms?

A cervical cap is pretty much just a smaller version of the diaphragm. It does have some important differences, however. First, it's smaller than a diaphragm and tightly covers the cervix and, second, it can be left in place for up to 36 hours.

A visit to the doctor is required to be fitted for the cervical cap. As with the diaphragm, it needs to be left in place for 6 hours after intercourse, but it should not be used during the woman's menstrual cycle.

There have been problems with cervical caps collecting secretions, causing inflammation of the cervix, and producing a highly unpleasant-smelling discharge. Also, its failure rate hovers around 16%. Cervical caps are not commonly used by women as a form of birth control, and my experience is that this particularly holds true for teenagers.

69. What is a contraceptive sponge?

A contraceptive sponge consists of polyurethane material that is saturated with a spermicide. It's considered both a physical and a chemical barrier method of birth control. A contraceptive sponge must be soaked in running water before it is inserted in the vagina, and then it needs to be left in place for 6 hours after intercourse.

There is an increased risk of yeast infections and bladder infections with the sponge, and if a woman leaves one in her vagina too long, there may be an increased risk of Toxic Shock Syndrome.

The sponge was very popular when it was first released in 1983, but then it was taken off the market in 1994 when it was learned that the water supply in the plant where the sponge was manufactured had become contaminated with bacteria. The sponge itself was never deemed unsafe. In 2005, it was reapproved for use by the FDA, and it's now readily available in drug stores.

That doesn't mean that contraceptive sponges are perfect, however. There is an increased risk of yeast infections and bladder infections with the sponge, and if a woman leaves one in her vagina too long, there may be an increased risk of Toxic Shock Syndrome. Also, the failure rates for the sponge are around 15%, and they don't provide STD protection.

When the sponge was initially released, I would periodically see patients to assist them in removing a sponge that had gotten wedged high up in their vaginas and they couldn't remove it by themselves.

70. What does my daughter need to know about birth control pills?

Hormonal contraceptive methods typically involve what we all refer to as birth control pills. One of their main mechanisms of preventing pregnancy is to prevent ovulation in the first place. Simply put, if there's no egg, it can't be fertilized. And if there's no fertilized egg, there's no baby.

Birth control pills also cause a woman's cervical mucus to thicken. That means that the man's sperm is less likely to be able to travel all the way to the woman's uterus. In addition, birth control pills cause the lining of a woman's uterus to become thinner. This makes it much more difficult for a fertilized egg to become firmly attached to the side of the uterus.

All of these mechanisms combined make the pill a very effective form of birth control. When used correctly the failure rate is 1%. However, typical use failure rates are around 5%–8%. Failures are usually the result of the woman forgetting to take the pills at the appropriate intervals. That's why, as double insurance, condoms should be used in addition to the pill. (And, as we discussed above, condoms should be used every time anyway as a means of decreasing the chances of contracting an STD.)

For the vast majority of healthy young women, the pill is perfectly safe. The main risk it poses stems from the effect of the estrogen in the pill, which can increase the risk of blood clots in the legs or pelvis. However, this increased risk is actually still lower than that typically experienced by women when they're pregnant.

This risk assessment isn't intended to minimize the effect of blood clots. On the contrary, they can be quite dangerous if they travel to the lungs, heart, or brain. Therefore, any woman who has an increased risk of blood clots should not take birth control pills. This particularly holds true for women who smoke. Research conclusively proves that they have a higher rate of blood clots, and this risk increases with age.

Any teenager or young adult I see who is on the pill and yet who still smokes has to listen to my friendly lecture on the hazards of tobacco. Needless to say, I strongly encourage these patients to stop smoking as soon as possible, and I offer them medical advice on how best to do so. Many young women defend their habit by telling me that they only smoke in social situations. However, it has been my observation that as I continue to see these patients over the years, the number of cigarettes they use increases—often substantially—over time. As I point out to them, quitting is much easier when you are only smoking a few cigarettes a day. The longer you wait to quit, the harder it is to quit.

The most common birth control pill in use today is a combination pill that contains both estrogen and progesterone hormones.

In addition to smokers, women with uncontrolled high blood pressure also should avoid birth control pills. Further, those who take them should realize that they face a small increased risk of gallbladder and liver problems.

The most common birth control pill in use today is a combination pill that contains both estrogen and

progesterone hormones. When birth control pills were first formulated decades ago, they typically contained high doses of estrogen. As a result, clotting problems were not uncommon. Over time, the estrogen dose in the pill has been lowered to safer levels.

The typical low-dose pill contains 30–35 ug of estrogen hormone, while the ultra-low-dose pill contains only 20–25 ug. The ultra-low-dose pill was originally intended for women in their forties, for women with high blood pressure that was well controlled, and for smokers. Now, however, the ultra-low-dose pill is the standard "first start" pill for young, healthy, non-smoking women, too.

Although the estrogen dose is lower, these ultra-low-dose pills have the same effectiveness as the standard low-dose pills, and importantly, they often have fewer side effects. When I start my patients on ultra-low-dose pills I mention that "breakthrough bleeding" (that is, bleeding that occurs in between menstrual cycles), may occur with more frequency. I tell them to call me if this is a persistent problem.

When birth control pills were first developed, scientists thought they had to mimic the normal menstrual cycle. Therefore, the pill packs contained 21 days of hormone pills and 7 days of **placebo** pills for a total of 28 pills. Patients were told that a pill needed to be taken each day and that their menstrual cycle would occur sometime during the placebo week. However, over time it became apparent that women didn't need to have a period once a month while taking the birth control pill. In fact, for many women a monthly period was nothing more than a nuisance and was accompanied by annoying symptoms such as cramping and headaches that could keep them

Birth Control

Progesterone

Progesterone is produced by the ovaries following ovulation and is responsible for preparing the lining of the uterus for pregnancy. When progesterone levels decline, menstruation occurs. Some of the side effects of progesterone include moodiness, headaches, acne, bloating, and depression. Synthetic forms of progesterone are found in hormonal methods of birth control.

Placebo

A substance that contains no medicine. "Sugar pills" found in packs of birth control pills are placebo pills.

from going to work or school. Thus was born the "continuous dosing" or "extended use" pill.

With the continuous dosing method, there are 91 pills per pack. The first 84 pills contain hormones and the last seven don't. A woman who follows this regimen has a period every 3 months during the placebo week of pills.

The purpose of including these seven placebo pills in the pack, rather than simply telling the woman to discontinue taking a pill for 7 days, is because it's important for women to establish a routine of taking the hormone pills each and every day so that they don't forget to do so. Further, it removes any doubt about when the woman is supposed to resume taking the hormones.

It's very important for the woman to ensure that there isn't any break between the end of using one pill pack and the beginning of using the next one. The failure to resume taking the hormone pills after 7 days of taking the placebo pills means that ovulation can occur. And *that* means the woman can become pregnant.

During a month that pills are taken late or are missed in their entirety, it's particularly prudent to use a backup birth control method such as condoms to ensure that pregnancy doesn't occur.

If a woman does forget to take a hormone pill, she should resume taking them immediately. Moreover, if need be, she should "double up" on the birth control pills the next day. During a month that pills are taken late or are missed in their entirety, it's particularly prudent to use a backup birth control method such as condoms to ensure that pregnancy doesn't occur.

There are some variations to the birth control regimen. For instance, some women opt to have periods even less frequently than once every 3 months. They can do so by continuously taking the hormone pills. However, it's important to note that there can be a significant initial incidence of breakthrough bleeding during the first 3 to 6 months.

Also, instead of placing pills in the pack that are strictly placebos, many manufacturers have begun adding low levels of hormones to the placebo-week pills. This step is designed to still permit a woman's monthly cycle to occur, but to reduce its related symptoms such as menstrual headaches.

Over the years I have come to the realization that there is no single type of birth control pill that is perfect for everybody. Some women like having a monthly cycle because it seems more natural and it reassures them that they're not pregnant. Other women see no point of putting up with the hassles of periods at all. Some women say that certain types of birth control pills make them moody. There are other pills that cause some women to experience skin outbreaks, and so on.

Because of these differences, your daughter should work closely with her doctor to determine which birth control pill is best for her. Further, your daughter should realize that the pill she is started on might not be the one that she eventually chooses for the long-term. Instead of stopping mid-cycle whenever they're taking a form of the pill that they decide they don't like, patients can call their doctor and switch to another type of pill without losing the contraceptive benefits of the hormones.

There's no doubt that the listed side effects of birth control pills are numerous. However, you and your daughter should know that the majority of females find these side effects to be minor in nature, and many of these side effects disappear after the first month.

Nevertheless, many women do initially experience some nausea and breast tenderness when they first begin using birth control pills. Although these symptoms should subside, if your daughter has persistent nausea, she should try taking the pill just before she goes to bed at night.

You and your daughter also should know that the benefits connected to taking the pill are numerous. For instance, the birth control pill decreases a female's risk of uterine and ovarian cancer. Moreover, even for those women with a family history of breast cancer but no other risk factors, most experts agree the pill does not increase their breast cancer risk.

The birth control pill decreases a female's risk of uterine and ovarian cancer.

Other benefits of the pill include a decrease in ovarian cysts and pelvic infections, a decrease in bone loss, less **fibrocystic breast disease**, an improvement of symptoms related to polycystic ovarian disease, less anemia (due to the fact that most women on the pill notice a lightening and shortening of their cycle), a decrease in the risk of infections spreading from the vagina up to the uterus and pelvis (because the hormones in the pill cause the cervical mucus to thicken), an improvement in pelvic pain due to **endometriosis** and ovulation, and less acne. I also use the pill for females who complain of moodiness or premenstrual syndrome, and I usually see an improvement.

Fibrocystic breast disease

A very common, benign disorder that arises before a menstrual cycle and encompasses a variety of symptoms such as breast tenderness, lumpiness, and discomfort.

Endometriosis

A disease that is characterized by abnormal implants of cells in the female pelvis that cause pain, adhesions, and infertility. Endometriosis can run in families and usually requires surgery to diagnose. It is often treated with the birth control pill but sometimes needs stronger medications or surgical treatment.

There is one quirk to birth control pills that you should be aware of. Specifically, a small percentage of women who discontinue using the pill may experience a delay of up to three months in ovulating. However, other women who discontinue using the pill may immediately become *extremely* fertile. This can be caused by the fact that when you take away the suppression effect of the pill, there can be a spike in the ovulation hormone, and therefore an egg can be released right away. In other words, you have the classic boomerang effect.

Another form of the birth control pill is the progestin-only pill, also formerly known as "POPs" or the "mini-pill." As the name indicates, this type of pill only contains the progesterone component and not any estrogen. This is a pill for women who cannot tolerate the side effects of estrogen, who may have hypertension, who have a history of blood clots, who smoke, or who are breastfeeding.

There are 28 hormone pills and no hormone-free pills in this type of pill pack. Progestin-only pills will not regulate cycles like the combination pill, and they work through the progesterone effect on the woman's cervical mucus and uterine lining. It is important for a patient to take these pills at the same time every day. If a woman is more than 3 hours late in doing so, then a backup method of birth control, such as a condom, needs to be used for at least 48 hours. However, if used correctly, the progestin-only pills have almost the same effectiveness as combination pills.

71. How does a vaginal ring work?

Vaginal rings are another form of hormonal birth control. They're similar to birth control pills because their contraceptive benefits are derived from estrogen and progestin. However, instead of taking the hormones by mouth as with pills, the hormones in the ring are absorbed directly through the vaginal wall when the woman places the ring in her vagina.

Vaginal rings are left in the vagina for three weeks, and then they are removed for one week. It's during that fourth week that a menstrual cycle occurs.

Vaginal rings are left in the vagina for three weeks, and then they are removed for one week.

The effectiveness of vaginal rings is similar to birth control pills. However, they have the added benefits of a very low rate of breakthrough bleeding, and the woman doesn't have to worry about remembering to take a pill every day. However, I tell my patients that they may notice some increase in their normal vaginal discharge.

Most partners won't notice the ring in the vagina during intercourse. However, if they do, and if it bothers them, the ring can be removed for up to 3 hours without losing its effectiveness.

72. Is the contraceptive patch safe and effective?

The patch consists of an adhesive swath of material containing estrogen and progestin that is affixed to the skin once a week. It's a convenient method of birth control for those women who don't want to take a daily pill, and its effectiveness is similar to the pill. However, the patch is currently under scientific scrutiny because there are some concerns that those women who use it might experience a higher incidence of blood clots.

73. How does Depo-Provera work?

Depo-Provera is progestin that is given to a woman via an injection. Depo-Provera has been around for years, and initially it required a visit to the doctor's office every 3 months for an intramuscular injection. However, a newer version has been developed that only requires a routine skin injection. This means that women can now be taught to give themselves the shot, or if they prefer, they can continue to go to the doctor's office for it.

Depo-Provera carries the same side effects as most hormonal methods. However, there are three additional points to keep in mind. First, when a woman begins using Depo-Provera, it's likely that her menstrual cycle will stop completely. Second, when a patient stops using it, her fertility may not return for several months. And third, Depo-Provera has been shown to cause some women to gain weight. In fact, the weight gain can be as much as 15 pounds. (You can imagine the looks I get each time I mention this fact to my patients.)

Nevertheless, it has to be noted that Depo-Provera is a highly effective form of contraception. When used correctly, the effectiveness is greater than 99%. Those are pretty good odds.

Depo-Provera is a highly effective form of contraception. When used correctly, the effectiveness is greater than 99%.

74. What is Implanon?

Implanon was approved by the FDA in 2006. It consists of a flexible rod the size of a matchstick that is placed under the skin of a woman's arm. (You usually can't see it after it's been implanted by a specially-trained health care provider.)

The Implanon rod contains only progestin, and therefore it carries with it the associated side effects of progestin that I mentioned previously. Moreover, it can only be removed in a doctor's office, and there can be persistent spotting and irregular bleeding with this method of birth control. However, Implanon's effectiveness is rated at greater than 99%, its contraceptive effects can last up to 3 years, and it doesn't require taking a pill daily.

75. What is emergency contraception?

Emergency contraception, also known as "the morning-after pill," is a type of hormonal birth control that's used to help prevent pregnancy when no method was used at the time of sexual intercourse, or when the method that *was* used failed (such as if the condom broke). As the term "emergency" implies, this method should not be used routinely as a means of birth control; its effectiveness at preventing pregnancy only ranges between 75%–89%. However, you have to admit that those odds are far better than merely keeping your fingers crossed.

Emergency contraception can consist of a combination pill or a progestin-only pill.

Emergency contraception can consist of a combination pill or a progestin-only pill. For those women 17 years or over, it's now available behind the counter in the form of a progestin-only pill known as "Plan B." For teens under 17 years old, getting it requires a prescription. Plan B consists of taking 2 progestin pills 12 hours apart and the newer Plan B One-Step combines the two doses into one pill.

Although it's called the morning-after pill, it is actually most effective when it's taken as soon as possible after unprotected intercourse. However, it can be taken up to 120 hours later. It works by preventing the release of an egg from the ovary, thereby preventing fertilization of the egg by the sperm. It's important to note that it will not interrupt an already developed pregnancy.

76. What are the different types of intrauterine devices (IUDs) available?

Intrauterine devices, commonly referred to as IUDs, have a long history of use. However, their popularity suffered in the 1970s because of the problems related to a particular kind of IUD known as the Dalkon Shield.

Due to a flawed design, the Dalkon Shield caused serious infections in some women, and it ultimately was removed from the market. Interestingly, within the United States all other types of IUDs suffered from the bad publicity related to this incident. Consequently, although many types of IUDs are commonly used in Europe, there are only two that are approved for use in the United States.

Today's IUDs are very safe when used appropriately, and they carry only a very small risk of pelvic infection. The IUDs come in various forms and are inserted directly into the woman's uterus to prevent the man's sperm from fertilizing the woman's egg. Insertion of an IUD is usually performed during the woman's menstrual cycle to ensure that the patient isn't pregnant at the time. There are strings attached to the IUD for easy removal.

Intrauterine devices are very effective. The pregnancy rate for women who use them is less than 1%. The two IUDs currently available in the United States are ParaGard and Mirena.

The two IUDs currently available in the United States are ParaGard and Mirena.

The ParaGard IUD contains a coil of copper and is inserted into the woman's uterus. It works by both deactivating sperm as they swim by, and by damaging or destroying the egg before it can be fertilized. ParaGard is effective for 10 years. I tell my patients that they may see some changes in their menstrual cycles if they use the ParaGard IUD as their birth control method, such as an increased menstrual flow and more **cramps**. Nevertheless, these symptoms usually aren't bad enough to cause patients to have the IUD removed. On a technical note, patients who have Wilson's Disease, which is a genetic inability to process copper, or if they have a copper allergy, can't use the ParaGard IUD.

The Mirena IUD contains progestin and works similarly to the progestin-only birth control pill. Specifically, it thins out the lining of the uterus making periods

Cramps

A popular term used to describe the pain and discomfort originating from the uterus during the menstrual cycle. Cramps are often described as a feeling of uncomfortable pressure in the lower abdominal or back area.

much lighter or even absent in women who use this device, and it thickens the cervical mucus so that sperm can't migrate from the vagina up into the uterus. The Mirena IUD is effective for 5 years. During that time it can have the beneficial effect of making a woman's periods lighter if she previously had very heavy ones. In fact, a common result of this IUD is that a woman's cycles may stop altogether due to the suppressive effect of progestin on the uterine lining. This effect isn't harmful and is completely reversible. However, I also tell all my patients receiving the Mirena IUD that some irregular bleeding can happen during the first 3 to 6 months.

Because of the progestin, certain possible side effects are listed in the instruction pamphlet for the Mirena IUD. These include headaches, bloating, depression, and moodiness. However, because the progestin is mostly confined to the uterus, I rarely have patients report that they notice these problems.

Regardless of which type of IUD is inserted, there are certain risks associated with their use. First, there is a very small risk that when the IUD is inserted, it will go through the wall of the uterus and into the abdominal cavity. If that happens, the IUD would need to be removed by a surgical procedure.

Second, although the risk of pelvic infection is very low, it is not zero, and pelvic infections have the potential to cause infertility. If I am counseling a young woman who desires an IUD, I emphasize that it is important to be in a mutually monogamous relationship to limit her exposure to STDs. The riskiest time for an infection is the month after insertion of the IUD because the procedure can transport bacteria from the vagina into the uterus. After that time, infection is unlikely in those patients who are at a low risk of contracting STDs.

77. *What are the permanent methods of contraception?*

Permanent methods of birth control typically are not appropriate for adolescents and young adults, except in highly unusual circumstances. Patients undergoing one of these procedures must fully realize that it takes away *forever* their ability to have children. And as the old saying goes, forever is a long, long time.

One type of permanent birth control is tubal ligation. This is a surgical procedure that needs to be performed in the hospital under general anesthesia. The purpose of tubal ligation is to block the fallopian tubes and prevent the sperm from reaching the egg. The effectiveness of this procedure is approximately 98%–99%.

Another type of permanent birth control is a vasectomy— and thankfully, the responsibility rests on the man with this one! The purpose of a vasectomy is to block the tubes that carry sperm to the semen. This is a surgical procedure just like tubal ligation, and the effectiveness is the same, but there are a few key differences. First, a vasectomy can be performed with less risk to the patient. Second, the procedure can be performed with just local anesthesia. And third, it can be performed in a doctor's office. What's not to like?

Just so you'll know, after the vasectomy is performed it's still necessary to use an alternative method of birth control for a few months to make sure the vasectomy was successful in blocking the tubes, and even if it was, to permit all the lurking sperm to completely disappear from the man's semen.

The final form of permanent birth control is Essure. Perhaps you've never heard of it because it is relatively new.

With Essure, small coils are snaked up through the vagina, into the uterus, and then into the fallopian tubes in order to cause permanent blockage. The effectiveness is greater than 99%. Advantages include fewer surgical risks, no general anesthesia, and the ability to have it performed in either a hospital or an office setting. Disadvantages include the 3-month wait time required after the procedure to ensure that it was effective and the radiological test required to confirm that the tubes are blocked.

PART NINE

The "Sexualization" of Young Girls

What is "sexualization"?

What does an adolescent think sex is?

Are girls engaging in sex at a younger age?

More . . .

Recently I came across an album that my grandmother created in 1916. It contains pictures of all the glamorous women she idolized as a teenager. It was fascinating to reach across almost a century of time and see the stars my grandmother tried to mimic as a girl. Their elaborate hairstyles and their restrictive dresses emphasize the distance we women have come in all those years.

And yet, at the same time, peering at that album also underscored just how much my grandmother and my young daughter have in common. Whether a girl was born at the beginning of the last century or at the dawn of this one, cultural role models invariably play a big role in her young life.

Today, of course, what those cultural role models represent is much different than in my grandmother's day. In long-ago eras, role models for girls typically accentuated being demure and proper. Needless to say, that's certainly not the case in the twenty-first century.

Sexualization

The American Psychological Association defines this term as including one or more of the following criteria: a person's value is determined solely by his or her sexual appeal or behavior; a person is held to a standard whereby only physically attractive people are deemed to be worthy sexual beings; a person is viewed only as a "thing" for another's sexual use; and/or sexuality is inappropriately imposed upon a person.

In many instances, that's a good thing. Modern girls need to have role models who are independent, creative, and assertive. But as mothers, we need to draw a line when it comes to the **sexualization** of young girls. In too many instances, the mass media and the mass marketers seem determined to create a pervasive image that even young girls are sexual creatures or should strive to be. That message is wrong, it's offensive, and it is emotionally unhealthy for our daughters.

Any mother who has doubts about the intent of some merchandisers only needs to go into "fashionable" clothing stores for girls. On the racks, customers will invariably see T-shirts with sexual innuendoes printed on them, hot pink push-up bras, low cut jeans, and belly-baring tops—

all in sizes for 7 to 10 year olds. And if anyone thinks this marketing strategy doesn't have an effect, they should consider the following: In 2003, **"tweens"** (that is, girls between the ages of 7 and 12) spent $1.6 million on thong underwear. (It would be interesting to know what the conversations are like in those households where the dad does the laundry and he makes an unwelcome discovery about his daughter's choice of underwear.)

Tweens
Refers to adolescents who are no longer considered "children," but who are not yet teenagers.

A few years ago, I watched a news story on TV about teens and the sexy clothing available to them. A mother was interviewed in a store as she shopped with her young daughter. The daughter was pressing her to buy a tight, low-cut shirt because many girls at her school were wearing them. The mother refused to buy it because she considered it inappropriate.

The reporter interviewed the daughter separately. The girl said she wanted to buy the shirt because there was so much peer pressure at school and she wanted to fit in. Interestingly though, after further questioning the girl admitted that she was relieved that her mother wouldn't let her buy such clothing because wearing it would make her feel vulnerable. She said it also made her feel better that she could go back and tell her friends that it was her mother's fault that she didn't wear "cool" clothes. That way, she didn't have to explain to her peers her true feelings about the clothing.

You and I need to keep that story in mind the next time we're on a shopping spree with our daughters.

78. What is "sexualization"?

In 2007, the American Psychological Association presented a "Report of the Task Force on the Sexualization of Girls." This task force was formed in response to an outcry by parents, child advocacy organizations, psychologists, and journalists who noted that the sexualization of girls by the media and others is an increasing phenomenon and is harmful to girls. Not surprisingly, in study after study researchers found that women were far more likely than men to be portrayed in the media in a sexual fashion. And importantly, of all women, young ones were targeted the most.

According to the Task Force Report, sexualization occurs when:

1. A person's value is determined solely by his or her sexual appeal or behavior;
2. A person is held to a standard whereby only physically attractive people are deemed to be worthy sexual beings;
3. A person is sexually objectified—that is, a person is viewed only as a "thing" for another's sexual use; and/or
4. Sexuality is inappropriately imposed upon a person.

Sexualization is hazardous to our daughters. It degrades them, it causes problems with their long-term self-esteem, and it can even dupe them into thinking of, and treating, their own bodies as simply objects of other people's gratification. This latter phenomenon, known as **"self-objectification,"** has been fully documented in a significant number of adolescent, and even pre-adolescent, girls. Not only can this problem result in severe emotional turmoil for a girl or woman, it can also serve as the primary reason why she engages in risky sexual behavior.

Sometimes the sexualization process can creep up on us without our realizing it. For instance, consider a

Self-objectification

The American Psychological Association uses this term to describe young women who learn to think of and treat their own bodies simply as objects of others' desires.

nationally known brand of dolls that is targeted to youngsters and includes such things as heavy make-up, miniskirts, fishnet stockings, and provocative expressions. Or consider a famous line of dolls that now comes in a "bling-bling" style complete with a halter-top and go-go boots. Or think about a chain of stores that promotes dressing up for young girls, but includes costumes that seem designed for a Las Vegas showgirl. Are these consumer items just innocent make-believe for our daughters, or do they sow harmful seeds in their minds? Ultimately, you have to decide what's right for your daughter. But do so with your eyes wide open.

79. What does an adolescent think sex is?

One way that the sexualization of girls has crept into our society is through the re-definition of what acts constitute sex. I think it's safe to say that when we were growing up, oral sex was definitely considered sex. But nowadays, oral sex is portrayed as being a harmless, pre-sexual form of physical contact between boys and girls. As a result, more and more girls are performing oral sex on more and more boys at younger and younger ages.

Some counselors and sexual behavior researchers estimate that about half of all students engage in oral sex by the time they reach high school. Moreover, they believe it's not uncommon for some students to begin this practice in seventh grade. At one school in Virginia recently, the principal learned about an "oral sex party" that took place outside of school with approximately 25 middle school students. Many of these students were on the honor roll.

Some counselors and sexual behavior researchers estimate that about half of all students engage in oral sex by the time they reach high school.

Local newspapers reported that once the principal found out about this "party," he notified the *girls'* parents so that they could take action. But the school took no action to notify the *boys'* parents so that the boys could be counseled or disciplined. When interviewed anonymously, the girls cited several reasons for their participation in this oral sex party. Specifically, they said they did it because they wanted to be accepted by the larger group of kids, because they liked the boy and wanted to please him, and because it was a way to experiment with a sexual act that wasn't really sex. (And interestingly, these middle schoolers thought of oral sex exclusively as having a girl perform fellatio on a boy, and not as having a boy perform oral sex on a girl.)

Brett says:

From my own experience, teenagers tend to think of oral sex and vaginal sex as very separate entities. When the word sex appears in a conversation, it is most likely referring to vaginal sex. It is very rare that the term "oral sex" is used within a teenager's vernacular, mostly due to the fact that the word sex is in the phrase. Furthermore, "sex" is often related to condoms, and when teenage girls perform fellatio they do not use a condom. By drawing a clear line between the two, the seriousness of oral sex has been seriously downplayed in teenagers' minds.

80. Are girls engaging in sex at a younger age?

What's clear from these statistics and stories is that girls are becoming sexually involved with boys at younger and younger ages. That means they're doing so before they're really prepared to deal with the physical, as well as emotional, repercussions. (Remember, if your daughter engages just in oral sex, it's true she can't get pregnant, but she most certainly can get a sexually transmitted disease.) One author who wrote about this topic recently said that parents assume that their child will start experimenting with sex at the same age as the parent did. Judy Mann said one good rule of thumb in this newly sexualized age is to subtract *four years* from that time, and then to begin discussions about sex with your daughter at this earlier age.

When it comes to talking to your daughter about sexual peer pressure, you really don't need to take a different approach than the one you use when discussing other types of peer pressure with her. You know the drill— emphasize to her that if her friends are genuine, they'll accept her for who she is and won't try to force her to do things she doesn't want to do. But be mindful of the fact that when it comes to preparing your daughter to actually *resist* peer pressure, your actions will make far more of an impression on her than your words.

PART TEN

Body Art

What should my daughter know about tattoos?

What should I know if my daughter says she
wants a body piercing?

What should I do if my daughter's piercing
site gets infected?

More...

Body art

A form of art expressed on the human body. Some examples include tattoos, piercings, scarification, branding, and pubic hair designing.

Body art, such as tattoos, body piercings, and pubic hair styling, doesn't appear to be just a passing fad. Therefore, as mothers of adolescent daughters, we need to know all about it.

81. What should my daughter know about tattoos?

In the course of examining my patients, something I've seen more and more frequently are tattoos. These tattoos come in all shapes, sizes, colors, and varieties—just like the women who sport them. And what's more, these tattoos are located in a lot of different locations on these women's bodies. In addition to the usual, expected spots such as the ankle, leg, arm, and chest, in some instances they appear where only the woman's most intimate partner—or her gynecologist—could ever see them. (Oh, and I guess the tattoo artist had a pretty good look as well.)

I have seen all kinds of tattoos: cartoon figures, names, logos, words, fruits, animals, portraits, and symbols of undetermined significance. Some are cute, some are odd, some are interesting, and some are downright obscene. I have seen some that are works of art, and some that look as if the tattoo artist was drunk, blind, or both.

The tattoo that I remember most was on a young woman who came to my obstetrics practice. She had a picture of Gumby prominently tattooed on her stomach. As her belly grew during her pregnancy, so did Gumby. That thing stretched and stretched and stretched. However, by the time the baby had been delivered, poor old Gumby was a wavy, streaky mess.

The history of tattoos is rather interesting. They've been around for thousands of years, but in recent centuries in Western cultures, their use has ebbed and flowed. Further, until the last couple of decades, they were confined almost exclusively to men. They were popular among patriotic soldiers in World War II, resurfaced as an antisocial symbol in the 1960s, became a rock star emblem in the 1970s, and then died out for a while before becoming a part of mainstream culture in the 1990s. Now, most people don't even think twice when they see someone with a prominent tattoo. In fact, it's been estimated that as many as 23% of all high school and college students have tattoos, and half of those tattooed students are women.

Adolescents say they get tattoos for a variety of reasons: as a form of decoration, as an effort to enhance self-identity, as a sign of rebellion against their parents and/or society, as a means of gaining peer acceptance, and as an indication of group membership (including gang membership). Some researchers claim there is a correlation between getting tattoos (and body piercings) and engaging in risky behavior such as underage sex, binge drinking, smoking, and illegal drug use.

However, a number of other researchers dispute this assertion. They claim that studies of young adults with tattoos and body piercings show that they are similar to their peers without body art in terms of positive family relationships, parental education, and religious involvement. In fact, in one high school study, more than 50% of the students with body art had A or B grades.

Before your adolescent daughter even thinks about getting a tattoo, there are certain things that you, and she, need to know.

Kama says:

My daughters and I are big fans of constant change. So, I agree with the thought that a henna or removable tattoo is the only way to go. If you don't want to wear the same nail polish color every day, why would you want to get a "forever" tattoo?

82. How are tattoos created?

First, it's important to know how tattoos are actually created. The process begins when the tattoo artist draws the design for the tattoo on the customer's skin. Then he cleans the area and applies a thin layer of a petroleum jelly-like substance to the site.

Nowadays, most professional artists use an electric tattoo gun when working on their creation. The bar of these "guns" can hold up to 14 needles that puncture the skin up to several thousand times a minute. The needles are dipped in different colored inks as desired, and when they pierce the skin they deposit the ink just a few millimeters deep.

As the tattoo gun punctures the skin, blood seeps from the wound and the artist wipes it away. Professional, reputable tattoo artists use one-time disposable containers for the ink, and they dispose of the needles after each client.

When the tattoo artist is finished, he applies an anti-bacterial solution and a bandage to the site. After 24 hours the customer can remove the bandage. However, after that point she should continue to keep the tattooed area clean and moist with the application of an antibiotic ointment. If a scab forms, she shouldn't pick at it.

Additionally, the customer shouldn't rub the tattoo or expose it to direct sunlight, petroleum jelly, or rubbing alcohol. Moreover, the customer shouldn't go swimming, soak the site, expose it to shower jets, or wear clothes that will irritate or adhere to it. (I bet you didn't know that tattoos were so delicate, did you?) The tattoo site will take approximately two weeks to heal.

83. Are tattoos regulated?

It's also important to know that the FDA does *not* regulate the process of tattooing or the use of tattoo inks. Instead, the actual practice of tattooing is regulated by local jurisdictions. Furthermore, as strange as it may seem, the tattoo pigments themselves are not approved for intradermal (that is, under-the-skin) use, and some pigments contain lead, mercury, and arsenic.

The FDA does not regulate the process of tattooing or the use of tattoo inks.

Some of the pigments in the ink are industrial grade and are actually suitable for use in automobile paint. While professional tattoo artists are regulated, amateurs are not, and they may use unconventional pigments such as charcoal ink or mascara. They also have been known to use pencils, pens, and sewing needles to apply the ink.

84. What can be the health effects of getting a tattoo?

You and your daughter should know about the complications that can arise from getting a tattoo. Infections such as Hepatitis B and C, and skin infections caused by *Staph* bacteria, can be transmitted through the use of non-sterile needles. And although it's never been documented, some health professionals feel that a person getting a tattoo runs the risk of acquiring HIV.

Also, if a tattoo is obtained from a non-regulated facility or artist, the recipient may not be able to donate blood

Non-infectious complications from getting a tattoo can include allergic reactions to the pigments, granulomas (or nodules) that form around the tattoo, and keloid formation.

Granulomas

Localized nodules of tissue that result from infection or injury.

Keloids

A scar that extends beyond the site of the original wound and can grow over time. These scars can be hereditary and occur more often in African Americans, Latinos, and Asians. They commonly occur around piercing sites.

for up to 12 months. That's because there's a risk that the recipient was exposed to a blood-borne infection.

Non-infectious complications from getting a tattoo can include allergic reactions to the pigments, **granulomas** (or nodules) that form around the tattoo, and keloid formation. **Keloids** are thick, wide scars that can form any time you traumatize your skin. And interestingly, there have even been some reports of people experiencing burning and swelling of their tattoos when they've undergone an MRI. This odd result has been attributed to the metal content in some tattoo pigments.

85. How can I make it safer for my daughter to get a tattoo?

You're probably wondering what you should do if, even after you provide her with all the information, your daughter still insists on getting a tattoo. Well, one thing you can do is make sure she goes to a professional, reputable, and clean tattoo facility. A big step in achieving this goal is ensuring that the tattoo artist is a member of the Alliance of Professional Tattooists (APT).

The APT is a nonprofit, educational organization founded in 1992 to address the safety and health issues of tattooing. Both the APT and the Society for Permanent Cosmetic Professionals (that permanent eyeliner you see on some women is a tattoo as well) have endorsed specific guidelines for their members to adhere to.

In addition, the APT has spelled out specific things that consumers should look for in determining whether a tattoo artist is following necessary safety procedures. Specifically, in addition to making sure that the tattoo shop is "clean like a medical facility," a potential customer should ensure that the tattoo artist always uses new needles that he removes from a sealed envelope, that he pours fresh ink into a new disposable container, and that he puts on new, disposable gloves before even beginning to set up his supplies.

86. Can tattoos be removed?

It's not uncommon for people to become dissatisfied with their tattoos, either because their tastes have changed or because the artist didn't do a particularly good job. (Also, you and your daughter should keep in mind that some job interviewers view prominent tattoos as a big turn-off.) Although removing tattoos is difficult, there are several options, such as laser treatments, dermabrasion (using a sanding disc), salabrasion (using a salt solution to essentially "scrub off" the tattoo), scarification (using acid to produce a scar to remove the tattoo), or camouflaging the area with skin-toned pigments. These methods of tattoo removal are neither cheap nor fun.

One way for your daughter to avoid the pain, expense, and hassle of getting or removing a permanent tattoo is to get a temporary or henna tattoo. Temporary tattoos are applied with moistened cotton and fade over several days. Henna tattoos last longer and are created by applying to the skin a dark, red-brown dye derived from the henna plant.

Most temporary tattoo dyes are approved for skin use. (Just watch out for foreign imports that are not FDA approved.) Henna is approved for hair dye use but not skin use. Allergic skin reactions can occur with both of these tattoo alternatives. All adverse reactions to permanent or temporary tattoos should be reported to the FDA. Your local FDA district office can be located in the blue pages of your local phone directory or by contacting the FDA's Center for Food Safety and Applied Nutrition (CFSAN) Adverse Events Reporting System (CAERS).

87. What should I know if my daughter says she wants a body piercing?

In addition to tattoos, body piercings have also become very popular among adolescents. One Canadian study found that more than half of all students with body piercings got their first one before the age of 15. While earlobes remain the most common site for piercings, just about any part of the body can be pierced. The following is a list of the most common sites—and some helpful medical tips that your daughter should keep in mind.

Nose—These piercings are usually done through the nostril, but they also can be done through the cartilage of the nasal septum, which can be very painful. Nose piercings can take 2 to 3 months to heal because of the poor circulation in the cartilage of the nose. Additionally, *Staph* bacteria commonly found in the nasal passages can be a source of infection.

Oral—The most common site for oral piercings is the lower lip, but sometimes people have their tongues pierced. When either of these sites is pierced they can become quite swollen. In fact, when the tongue is pierced you have to put a long bar in place initially to accommodate the swelling. This bar is then replaced with a shorter one once the swelling subsides. Further, tongue piercings have been documented to cause enough swelling in a person's mouth to lead to airway obstruction. Other complications can include tooth fractures, tooth chipping, interference with chewing and swallowing, increased salivation, infection, loss of taste, speech difficulty, numbness, and inhalation of jewelry.

Tongue piercings have been documented to cause enough swelling in a person's mouth to lead to airway obstruction.

Tongue piercings take 1 to 2 months to heal, while lip and cheek piercings can take 3 to 4 months.

Facial—This site is usually the eyebrow, which should be pierced on the outer part, away from the bridge of the nose. This is a common piercing site for men, and it poses relatively few difficulties.

Ear—In addition to the lobe, which is the most common and perhaps safest place to be pierced, the auricle (or rim) of the ear can also be pierced. Because of the poor blood supply in the cartilage of the ear, healing can take 3 to 4 months.

Navel—This site is very common among girls, but it also seems particularly susceptible to infections, such as from *Staph* bacteria. The piercing should always be done on the skin above the navel, and protruding belly-buttons can make this piercing difficult. This site typically takes 4 to 6 months to heal.

Nipple—The nipple is usually pierced horizontally, but it can be done vertically. Nipple piercing usually doesn't interfere with breastfeeding as long as the mother remembers to take out the jewelry before the child starts nursing. This site usually heals in 4 to 6 months, but sometimes breast abscesses occur.

Genital—Females can have their labia or clitoris pierced. These sites can take 1 to 4 months to heal. Piercing of the clitoris can cause fibrosis (or thickening) of that highly sensitive part of the female anatomy, and piercing behind the clitoris is risky because it can compromise the blood flow.

The healing times I've cited for different piercing locations are averages. Sometimes, complete healing in certain sites can take up to a full year.

Jewelry for piercing should be made of surgical-grade stainless steel, titanium, niobium, solid platinum, or 14K or 18K gold to help prevent a reaction. A plastic such as Tygon can be used as well.

88. How should the ear piercing process work?

Because earlobe piercing is the most common type of body art for adolescent girls, I'll focus on that process.

Typically when a girl gets her ears pierced, a piercing gun is used. As the gun shoots the earring stud into the girl's earlobe, the tissue of the ear is torn. This compares to the earlobe being surgically cut with a needle as professional piercers do. The gun is often described as a more painful experience.

Piercing guns should only be used for lobes and not for the rim of the ear or any other body part.

Piercing guns should only be used for lobes and not for the rim of the ear or any other body part. The older piercing guns were hard to completely clean, let alone sterilize, but disposable, sterile cartridges have now been designed with a sterile earring in it for one-time use. However, many piercing professionals oppose all types of piercing guns. They state that there is no way to effectively sterilize the entire unit regardless of the sterile cartridge, and that the guns can crush tissue and result in embedded earrings and earring backs that may have to be surgically removed.

Kama says:

You know the drill. You've reluctantly capitulated and gotten your daughter's ears pierced. At first she is content with the tiny adornments in her new stylishly clad lobes but it doesn't last long and inevitably she has to have hoops. All the other girls and some of the boys are wearing them, and reportedly, she looks like a baby.

So what do you do? Give in? Before you do, remember that the dog jumps up on her when she walks in the door and unless your pooch is a mini, there is a real possibility that the dog will be wearing the new hoop earrings as paw rings. Don't have a dog? What about a roughhousing sibling? A torn ear lobe is a torn ear lobe, no matter how it happens. You will wish you'd stuck to your guns and your daughter will too.

89. Are professional piercers regulated?

Just like tattoo artists, professional piercers have created an organization dedicated to the health, education, and safety of piercers and the public. The Association of Professional Piercers (APP) requires its members to have at least one year of piercing experience, be trained in cardiopulmonary resuscitation and blood-borne pathogens, and have a current first-aid certificate. Further, the APP requires its members to get written parental consent before performing any procedure on a minor, and it considers nipple or genital piercings to be inappropriate for anyone younger than 18.

The APP recommends that before anyone undergoes a piercing procedure, he or she should check whether the piercing facility meets certain criteria, to include the following:

Use of a medical-grade autoclave with spore testing to ensure that all instruments have been properly sterilized;

Use of individually wrapped sterile needles that are not reused;

Use of piercing methods other than piercing guns;

Use of new disposable gloves;

Availability of a diverse jewelry selection for the specific body part to be pierced;

Presentation of an "after-care" sheet to clients;

Licensing, if required, by local or state regulators; and

Membership in the APP by the person doing the piercing.

I think all of these recommendations are good ones and should be closely followed by anyone getting an oral, navel, genital, nipple, or facial body piercing. However, when it comes to simple earlobe piercing, good, clean, well-managed jewelry shops at local malls should work out just fine, even though they're not approved by the APP. Thousands and thousands of people get their ears pierced at these types of stores every year, and there doesn't seem to be much of a problem.

I recently went to a nearby shopping mall and visited a store that pierces ears to see exactly how the process works. The mother of the girl who was getting her ears pierced first had to sign a consent form. Then the employee washed her hands and put on a pair of new, clean vinyl gloves from a box. She next wiped the plastic piercing gun handle with alcohol swabs. She then wiped the girl's earlobes in the front and back with another alcohol pad and marked the earlobe-piercing site with a marker.

The employee next opened a package containing a sterile cartridge with a sterile earring and, without touching it, loaded the cartridge into the gun handle. When the employee pierced the girl's earlobe, only the sterile cartridge came in contact with her earlobe. The cartridge was then released and discarded. The girl winced when her earlobe was actually pierced, but she didn't seem to be in much pain. As a final step, the employee of the store provided the girl's mother with an after-care kit.

Of course, the entire experience hinges on the person doing the piercing. If your daughter is getting her ears pierced, you may want to call ahead and ask when the store's most experienced person is going to be working.

90. What should I do if my daughter's piercing site gets infected?

If your daughter gets her ears pierced and an infection results, she should try to leave the jewelry in place during treatment. Removal of the jewelry may lead to closure of the piercing site and may also prevent the infection from draining properly. This can lead to an abscess. In most instances, all that will be needed is for your daughter to apply warm compresses to the infected area and to wash the site with an antibacterial soap. Topical ointments are not recommended. Oral antibiotics and, rarely, intravenous antibiotics may be necessary in certain circumstances where the infection doesn't resolve itself.

To reduce the risk of infection or other complications such as bruising, scarring, and keloid formation, your daughter should take certain steps if she gets a body piercing.

Generally speaking, for non-oral sites she should soak the area in a saltwater solution 2 or 3 times a day and wash it with an antibacterial soap 1 to 2 times a day. She should not use alcohol, hydrogen peroxide, Betadine, Hibiclens, or ointment on the area. She should prevent any bumping, jostling, or rubbing of the site, and she should avoid pools and hot tubs until the piercing has healed. When she takes a shower or bath, she should cover the piercing with a waterproof bandage.

And finally, she should leave the jewelry in place for the entire healing process.

For nipple piercings, your daughter should wear a tight cotton shirt or a sports bra. This clothing provides protection and support, and it won't rub back and forth against the jewelry.

For navel piercings, a woman should cover the area with a hard, vented eye patch to provide protection from clothing and irritation.

For genital piercings, a woman should use barriers such as condoms during sex to protect against her partner's body fluids. Only a water-based lubricant from a new container should be used during intercourse. The site should be soaked in saline or rinsed in clean water after any sexual contact. If the piercing is near the woman's urethra, she should urinate after she cleans the area with soap.

For oral sites, during the entire healing process a woman should rinse her mouth 4 to 5 times a day for 30 to 60 seconds using an antimicrobial/antibacterial, alcohol-free mouth rinse or a package of sterile saline solution. For the first few days after piercing, she will need to avoid hot, spicy, salty, or acidic foods.

91. What should my daughter know about pubic hair removal and styling?

Another trend that has become quite widespread among adolescents and teens is pubic hair removal or styling. In fact, some girls start removing their pubic hair as soon they notice it growing in. Girls as young as 11 and 12 years old are showing up in their doctor's office with pubic razor stubble. Typically these girls have learned about this practice by seeing or reading about hair removal products or pubic hair grooming in magazines or the Internet, or by hearing about it from an older sister or friend. Often Mom is the last to know and only finds out when the adolescent has injured herself with Dad's sharp razor.

As discussed in the hygiene section, trimming, shaving, or bikini-waxing pubic hair is very common among adolescents. But some go so far as to get Brazilian-style bare waxing, which means complete removal of all pubic hair, or to dye their pubic hairs different and unusual colors, or to style their pubic hairs in different shapes, sometimes using stencils.

If she feels that she needs to, there are several ways your daughter can remove pubic hair. Shaving with a razor is the most common, followed by waxing. Laser hair removal is now offered by many medical offices and, in experienced hands, provides good results. **Depilatories** are chemical substances and are another common method of pubic hair removal. These products are available over the counter.

Although many females remove hair without a problem, sometimes the following complications can be seen.

Razor Burn—This can be caused by shaving dry skin, making too many passes over the skin, or by using a dull blade. There are many safer versions of razors for women available in drugstores. Razor burn can be treated with a mild steroid cream and moisturizers.

Folliculitis—This is an inflammation and/or infection of the hair follicle and can be seen with many of the pubic hair removal methods. *Mechanical folliculitis* is

Depilatories

Products such as creams, lotions, and powders that contain chemicals that remove hair. These products are commonly used to remove pubic hair and leg hair and are available over the counter.

Folliculitis

Inflammation of the hair follicle. Folliculitis can be painful and is caused by skin bacteria. It is often seen in the pubic hair region and appears as small pimple-like structures. Folliculitis can occur from the use of hair removal products, shaving, or waxing.

117

inflammation without infection and is caused by hairs that don't grow back straight, usually after using a blade or waxing. Both a steroid cream and a topical antibiotic cream can be used for a few days after shaving to help prevent folliculitis, but if this is a persistent problem, it may be necessary to switch to a safety razor, an electric razor or trimmer, or laser hair removal. *Infectious folliculitis* is when there is an actual infection of the hair follicle and pimples appear. The infection is often caused by common skin bacteria, such as *Staph* and *Strep*, and may need antibiotic treatment to resolve.

Spread of Infection—This can occur with shaving, waxing, and depilation. Because these methods cause injury to the skin, they allow bacteria to enter. Just as with shaving, they can enhance the spread of infection over the surfaces involved. These infections include skin bacteria as well as herpes, molluscum contagiosum, and HPV. Adolescents have been known to shave their pubic hair in order to get a better look at genital warts or molluscum bumps, only to spread the infection even further.

Contact Dermatitis—Any product used on the delicate skin of the genital area can cause a painful or itchy reaction. This can be treated by stopping use of the product, accompanied by gentle cleansing of the area and use of a steroid cream. Depilatories, which are creams that contain chemicals that dissolve the hair, should only be used on the bikini line area and nowhere else because they can cause extreme irritation and skin burns.

PART ELEVEN

Other Issues Affecting Your Daughter

What should I know about eating disorders?

What are some of the more common psychological issues seen in adolescent females?

How common is alcohol abuse among adolescents?

More . . .

I'm not a mental health professional. My medical specialty is obstetrics and gynecology. But as a physician who sees hundreds and hundreds of patients each year, I've always considered it my professional responsibility to guide women, both young and old, so that they will seek the emotional, psychological, or psychiatric treatment or counseling they may need. As a mother, it's vitally important for you to also assume this role when it comes to your daughter.

As you well know, the adolescent years for your daughter are likely to be filled with excitement, fun, turmoil, angst, and melodrama. That's perfectly normal. Hormones can go on a rampage at that point in a girl's life, and you may serve as a hapless bystander to their emotional mugging of your daughter. And yet, as she grows into adulthood, you're also likely to see that she has emerged relatively unscathed from this exasperating and exhilarating period of her life.

But at times, there are deeper and more powerful issues at work. When that's the case, we owe it to our daughters to do our best in ensuring that they receive whatever assistance or treatment they need, and that they get it as soon as possible.

I realize that this fact places a significant burden on you. When it comes to mental health issues, you're probably not an expert. However, when it comes to your daughter, there is no greater expert in the world. Therefore, as a mom, if you keep your eyes open, your mind open, and your heart open, you're likely to recognize when something is not quite right. Nonetheless, sometimes girls will be very diligent and effective at hiding these types of problems, particularly from those closest to them. As a result, sometimes a mother is the last person to know. But if you think there may be a problem, you need to get involved.

If you begin to believe that your daughter is experiencing emotional problems, talk to a school counselor; your daughter's pediatrician; your own doctor; or your local, city, county, or state mental health service. Tell them what you've observed and what your concerns are. They either will provide you with the reassurance you need that your daughter is perfectly fine, or they will help you find the help your daughter needs.

Unfortunately, even in the twenty-first century, there is an unfair stigma attached to mental health problems. But please don't let that fact stop you, or even delay you, from seeking assistance. Although not as visible as cuts and bruises, emotional problems can be even more harmful and debilitating to your daughter. If there is any point in a girl's life when she needs your help, this is it. Counselors and other mental health professionals can do wonders with young people. Don't hesitate to seek their assistance.

I've written this chapter to help you identify when your daughter may need psychological help. In doing so, I haven't prepared an exhaustive list of emotional issues and warning signs. I'm not sure anyone could. However, my hope is that the following pages will provide you with the information you need so that you can be alert to some of the most common problems that may arise. What you do with this information could make all the difference in the life of your daughter.

92. What should I know about eating disorders?

Although they can arise in either gender and at any age, eating disorders most commonly appear in females between the ages of 12 and 25. In fact, millions

Eating disorders most commonly appear in females between the ages of 12 and 25.

of young women suffer from anorexia and bulimia each year.

Parents often think that their daughter will grow out of the problem, or that they can independently help their daughter get past it. However, don't be tricked into inaction. The most effective way to treat an eating disorder is by getting a trained medical professional involved.

An eating disorder is typically caused by deep, underlying psychological problems that need to be addressed in order for a girl to recover from this affliction. And the seriousness and effects of such a problem shouldn't be minimized. Eating disorders can cause serious health complications, and even death, as we all saw with the singer Karen Carpenter.

Anorexia nervosa

An eating disorder where the patient has an abnormal perception of her body as being too fat. Extremely low body weight, self-starvation, and excessive exercise are commonly seen in patients with this disease. Professional psychiatric help is essential for treatment of this disorder.

Anorexia nervosa is a specific eating disorder that involves an obsessive preoccupation with dieting and thinness that causes a girl to literally starve herself. Girls who are particularly susceptible to anorexia are those who have low self-esteem and negative feelings about their bodies, those who enter puberty early, and those who participate in activities such as gymnastics or dancing where size and weight are important factors to success, and where others constantly emphasize that fact.

There are a number of warning signs for anorexia:

- An obsession with one's body weight;
- A distorted and baseless perception that one is overweight;
- An irrational desire to lose weight;
- Becoming anxious at mealtime;
- Secretly disposing of food rather than eating it, or only pretending to eat food in the presence of others;
- Avoiding social activities that involve food;

- Less regular menstrual periods;
- Exercising excessively;
- Binging on food and then purging it (see bulimia).

Chronic starvation of this nature can be highly dangerous. A girl's body can become malnourished, and then as it searches for calories and nutrients, organs begin to shut down and muscles begin to break down, including the heart muscle.

Bulimia nervosa is a different type of eating disorder. It typically involves frequent binging and purging, but the young woman who has this disorder may not be unusually thin. Oftentimes a girl who has bulimia has intense feelings of guilt or shame about food. A person with bulimia feels out of control but recognizes that her behavior isn't normal. It's estimated that up to 5% of all college women in the United States are bulimic.

The warning signs for bulimia include:

- Eating large amounts of food, usually in secret (binging);
- Vomiting or using laxatives excessively to rid the body of the increased calories (purging);
- Spending long periods of time in the bathroom after meals;
- Obsessing over one's weight;
- Having irregular periods;
- Suffering from mood swings; and
- Experiencing an erosion of tooth enamel caused by the acid in vomit.

I personally witnessed someone with bulimia when I worked near a beach after my first year of medical school. I rented a room in a house with several other people. One of the renters was a beautiful, blonde,

Bulimia nervosa
An eating disorder characterized by consuming large amounts of food, known as binging, and then getting rid of the food, or purging, through vomiting, laxative use, or with diuretics. Those affected are usually of normal weight. Professional psychiatric help is essential for treatment of this disorder.

normal-weight young woman who was working at the shore for the summer like me. She was very friendly, but she always seemed to avoid eating with the rest of us. She also spent a long time in the bathroom, but no one gave it much notice.

As the summer went on, her behavior became more erratic with bouts of moodiness. One day she just disappeared, without paying her share of that month's rent. When her family was contacted, they disclosed that the young woman had a history of bulimia. Further, when we cleaned out her room, we discovered trash bags full of empty jars of peanut butter and mayonnaise. (High-fat foods like these are used by bulimics to coat their GI tract so that when they vomit, the acid from their stomachs won't irritate their esophagus and throat.) We were all shocked by our discovery. My housemates just kept on commenting on how "normal" the young woman seemed. But I knew that this woman was desperately in need of help.

When it comes to eating disorders, the key to recovery is early diagnosis and professional help.

When it comes to eating disorders, the key to recovery is early diagnosis and professional help. There are many Internet sources that can guide you in finding the necessary assistance. A few include the National Association of Anorexia Nervosa and Associated Disorders, the National Eating Disorders Association, the Academy for Eating Disorders, and the National Institute of Mental Health.

Kama says:

While seeking professional help is the best course of action, once a young person shows signs of self-abuse, there may be some preventive measures that can be taken. As a former anorexic, I am only too familiar with its devastating effects, and it has been my fervent mission to protect my own children from this insidious affliction.

Usually, anorexia starts as a plan to diet. Women are bombarded on a daily basis with the social belief that in order to be of value, one must be young, thin, and beautiful on the outside. Therefore, even children, at a young age, learn about dieting as a means to achieve "perfection." We owe it to our daughters to help dispel this erroneous social expectation.

While I am not proposing that you deviate from a healthy lifestyle, I ask you to remember that you are your daughter's role model. Make it a point to never discuss your own weight or comment on the weight of others. Go one further. Toss out the bathroom scale. That single act will help demonstrate to our daughters that we judge ourselves and others by the beauty within.

93. What is "cutting"?

"**Cutting**" has received increased attention in recent years. It is a form of self-mutilation where girls literally cut their skin with knives, razors, or other sharp objects, and it is performed in a horribly misguided attempt to relieve extreme emotional stress. Adolescents who have "cut" say that it is their way of trying to convert emotional pain into physical pain that will eventually subside.

Some young people cut just to experience the act and never cut again. Others become addicted to the ritual for years. Those who repeatedly cut tend to have a higher likelihood of experiencing emotional problems, engaging in drug abuse, having endured prior sexual abuse, having an underlying eating disorder, exhibiting poor coping skills and self-esteem, lacking a good support system, and engaging in risky sexual practices such as unprotected intercourse.

Cutting

The practice of self-mutilation that involves cutting the skin with a sharp object in an attempt to ease internal pain, stress, or conflict. Typically the sites that are cut are hidden from view under clothing.

One warning sign to parents is when an adolescent has unexplained injuries on her arms or legs, or when she habitually wears long sleeves in warm weather to hide the cuts. Accompanying signs can include a change in behavior, friendships, and school performance. Burning, scratching, picking skin, pulling hair out, eye pressing, and biting are other forms of self-mutilation.

Any suspicion of self-mutilation warrants a visit to a professional trained in dealing with this practice such as a mental health therapist, psychologist, or psychiatrist and should be addressed immediately. Individual and group therapies and medication have been used successfully to treat this addictive habit.

94. What are some of the more common psychological issues seen in adolescent females?

Anxiety

Anxiety disorders are the most common mental health problem in adolescents.

Every child experiences some anxiety. It can range from showing intense distress when the child is separated from her parents, or normal short-lived fears of such things as the dark or thunderstorms or animals. However, children with an anxiety disorder have a much more pronounced problem. Their anxiety interferes with their daily life. They are overly worried about things and events, and they are constantly seeking reassurance from others.

Adolescence

The period of time from the onset of puberty to maturity. The World Health Organization defines this period of time as including ages 10–19. Other organizations include the ages of 8–21.

Anxiety disorders are the most common mental health problem in adolescents. Approximately 25% of adults have some form of such a disorder, and many state that their fears started in **adolescence**. A child's anxiety disorder can manifest itself in a host of ways, to include an obsessive fear about the safety of loved ones, a refusal to go to school, frequent stomachaches and physical complaints, excessive worrying about sleeping away from home, panic attacks or tantrums, being overly clingy, and having trouble sleeping.

Phobias

Phobias are intense fears about specific things that cause extreme distress and interfere with daily activities. Examples include an unshakeable fear of needles, animals, bees, fire, lightning, and so on.

Social Anxiety

Social anxiety includes the fear of meeting and interacting with people. It often results in avoidance of social situations.

Obsessive Compulsive Disorder

Obsessive compulsive disorder, which is also referred to as OCD, often is the product of, or the source of, significant levels of anxiety. It includes repetitive, unwanted thoughts called obsessions, and repetitive, unnecessary actions called compulsions. When people think of OCD, they often think of repetitive hand washing. But the truth is that OCD can manifest itself in many ways.

Simply telling your daughter to stop worrying about her obsessions or to stop engaging in her compulsive behavior will be of no use. If she could stop on her own she would. She needs professional help in order to attain that goal.

All of these anxiety disorders are seen frequently in children, adolescents, and young adults, and the only truly effective approach is early diagnosis and treatment. Recent studies have shown that many of these disorders can be controlled with behavioral therapy, sometimes in conjunction with medication. Ignoring the problem only embeds the anxiety disorder more deeply into the lives of children, and these young people then carry it into adulthood. Therefore, if your daughter shows signs of suffering from one of these problems, take her to a mental health professional.

Depression

It is estimated that approximately 5% of children and adolescents suffer from depression at some time. Those at higher risk are children who are under stress; who have experienced a loss; or who have attention, learning, behavioral, or anxiety disorders. There is also a tendency for depression to run in families.

Kama says:

My daughter was especially anxious over copious amounts of homework. After a long day at school, she often felt incapable of tackling 25–30 math problems. My solution was this: I would instruct her to complete the first five problems and then report back to me. I would stress that it must be five. No more. No less.

By taking control and dividing her task into a more easily attainable goal, her stress was diminished. When she had completed the five problems, I would then instruct her to do a silly physical activity (the sillier the better).

An example: Instruct her to walk from point A to point B with a book on her head, one finger on her nose and one finger on her foot (if she drops the book, she must start all over), or to go outside and run around the house . . . backwards . . . two times.

"But Mom . . . it's raining."

"You're right it is. Here's your raincoat."

These activities gave the OTHER side of her brain a challenge and were guaranteed to get both of us laughing. (It is true. Laughter is the best medicine.)

Consequently, I was able to instruct her to do several more questions, perhaps eight or nine, before her next "task." In so doing, she was able to complete all the homework, learn to reduce her stress, and even have some fun.

95. What are the warning signs for depression in my adolescent?

The depressed adolescent is different from the depressed adult in some ways. As noted by the American Academy of Child and Adolescent Psychiatry, you should look for the following warning signs in your daughter:

- Frequent sadness, tearfulness, and crying
- Decreased interest in previously favorite activities
- A sense of hopelessness
- Persistent boredom and low energy
- Social isolation and poor communication
- Low self-esteem and a misplaced sense of guilt
- Extreme sensitivity to rejection and failure
- Difficulty with relationships
- Frequent vague physical ailments, such as headaches and stomachaches
- Frequent absences from school or unexplained poor academic performance
- Poor concentration
- Major changes in eating or sleeping patterns
- Talk of, or efforts to, run away
- Unusual acts of misbehavior
- Comments about suicide, death, or self-destructive behavior

Because early diagnosis and treatment is essential, you should seek help for your daughter immediately if you suspect she has depression. Treatment of this disease can often be quite effective.

Kama says:

It isn't always easy to communicate with your teen. Sometimes it seems that you've lost your connection. How do you keep the lines of communication open even when your daughter is experiencing the rollercoaster that is adolescence? The answer may be quite simple.

I suggest an after-supper stroll . . . just the two of you. You may be pleasantly surprised that after the first few nights, you and she find that words, which somehow wouldn't come while sitting face to face, flow while on a walk. Sharing thoughts and feelings will keep you in tune with your daughter and solidify the fact that she can always come to you with her problems.

96. What should I know about the risks of suicide in adolescent girls?

Suicide is the third-leading cause of death among youth from 15 to 24 years of age.

Suicide is undoubtedly every parent's worst nightmare. Recently the CDC issued a report that noted suicide is the third-leading cause of death among youth from 15 to 24 years of age, and the fourth-leading cause of death among children from 10 to 14 years of age. In these age groups, the most common methods of suicide consist of firearms, hanging/suffocation, and poisoning.

Although there had been declining rates previously, the incidence of suicide from 2003 to 2004 increased for females from 10 to 14 years of age, and from 15 to 19 years of age. (However, males still account for about three-fourths of the adolescent and young adult suicides.)

To put this in hard numbers, in 2004 almost 450 girls between the ages of 10 and 19 committed suicide.

Recently there have been reports of unintentional asphyxia fatalities resulting from adolescents playing the "choking game." This "game" consists of a person intentionally restricting the supply of oxygen to the brain of herself or someone else in order to induce a brief sense of euphoria. Some of these tragic, unintentional fatalities may have been incorrectly listed as suicides.

Other speculation about the rise in the number of adolescent suicides involves the increased pressure of modern life on our young people, stiffer competition to make good grades, more violence in the media, and a lack of parental interest. Some young people reported that when they tried to tell their parents about their feelings of unhappiness or failure, the parents didn't take them seriously. Similarly, those who work with at-risk youth say that teens often make direct statements regarding their intent to end their lives, or indirect comments about how they would be better off dead, but they're ignored.

Please, please do not let a cry for help from your daughter go unheeded. Instead, be vigilant for the following warning signs as cited by the New York University Child Study Center:

- A change in eating and sleeping habits
- A marked personality change, such as exhibiting angry actions or rebellious behavior, or withdrawing from friends and regular activities
- Involvement in drugs or alcohol or other risky behaviors such as reckless driving
- An overreaction to a humiliating experience
- Difficulty in concentrating and a decline in the quality of school work

- Persistent boredom and lethargy
- Unusual neglect of her personal appearance
- Complaints about physical symptoms such as headaches and fatigue
- A pattern of giving away or throwing away possessions
- Intolerance of praise or rewards
- Preoccupation with death in writings, songs, or poems
- An increase in comments such as "I can't take it anymore," or "Nobody cares about me, I wish I were dead"

If you have any reason to believe that your daughter is having suicidal thoughts, you should contact a mental health professional immediately. In making your determination, take any comments she may make about self-hate, suicide, or death very seriously. If her statements seem indirect, ambiguous, or unclear, ask her about them. Don't be afraid to say the word "suicide." It won't put improper thoughts in her head, and it may reassure her that you've heard her cries for help.

If your daughter is depressed or has suicidal thoughts, don't try to convince her that she shouldn't feel bad, get angry about the situation, or tell her that she should "just snap out of it." It won't help, and it could in fact make things worse by making her feel even more frustrated and guilty about the fact that she feels the way she does. Instead, reassure her that you love her and that you are willing to work with her to address her problem. Then tell her that you're contacting someone who is skilled in helping young people wrestle with this problem, and do so.

97. How common is alcohol abuse among adolescents?

I don't think any parent nowadays needs to be told that a lot of teens are participating in underage drinking.

Experimentation with alcohol is common during adolescence. Teens have ready access to it in their homes, through older friends, or at parties. Many have watched their parents have a beer or a drink without adverse consequences, and they conclude that warnings about underage drinking are dramatically overblown. Furthermore, there's an awful lot of peer pressure to begin drinking at a young age.

In reality, however, underage drinking poses a large and serious problem. Many young people underestimate the effects of alcohol, and as a consequence, there are more than 10,000 alcohol-related motor vehicle deaths and 40,000 injuries each year. Further, young people are far more likely to engage in binge drinking, and the resulting acute levels of alcohol in the bloodstream can cause real damage to their brains and bodies. In fact, asphyxiation on vomit is a real risk, as is alcohol poisoning, which leads to death. And finally, some researchers believe that drinking at an early age increases the risk that a person will develop an addiction later in life and leads to use of other drugs.

By 1998, all states had adopted a minimum alcohol purchase and drinking age of 21. In spite of this—and some critics of these laws would argue, because of this—in 2007, 26% of high school students reported periodic binge drinking. In response, some parents have decided to host parties in their home where alcohol use by high school kids is allowed. These parents seem to feel that by taking this action, they are reducing the chances that their kids will be on the roads while either they, or their friends, are under the influence of alcohol.

Needless to say, however, these parents need to ask themselves whether this truly is the best approach to

Other Issues Affecting Your Daughter

133

addressing the problem of underage drinking. They also need to realize that they are putting themselves in legal jeopardy. Just recently in Virginia, a mother who sponsored a party in her home where alcohol was freely served to teenagers was sent to prison for a number of months.

Drinking is a serious matter. You need to talk to your daughter about it, and you need to tell her directly about your views and expectations.

Brett says:

It is a natural part of high school and adolescent development to be confronted with the consumption of alcohol. I have personally had two experiences with alcohol abuse where fellow students ended up in the hospital. However, it is more important to learn from these mistakes than to focus on the illegality of drinking. It is important that teenagers understand that they have options if they ever drink and find themselves in a difficult position. I am lucky enough to have parents that understand the difficulties of peer pressure in high school and trust me enough to make the right decisions. Most importantly, my parents have given me the opportunity to call them in any situation if there is no sober driver.

98. What are the more common forms of drug abuse among adolescents?

Marijuana is the most commonly used illegal drug, and the average age of first use is 14.

In addition to alcohol, teens abuse many other drugs, both legal and illegal. Marijuana is the most commonly used illegal drug, and the average age of first use is 14. Other common drugs are cocaine, LSD, PCP, opiates, heroin, and designer drugs like ecstasy. In fact, the daughter of a good friend of mine told me recently that cocaine use is not uncommon in her high school, a high-achieving school in a very well-to-do area.

Abuse of prescription medications and over-the-counter medicines is also quite high among youths. The most commonly abused ones are pain relievers, tranquilizers, stimulants, and depressants. Cough and cold medicines seem to be a particular favorite. In addition, it's estimated that more than 2 million teens abuse prescriptions medications each year.

Drug use can have serious negative consequences, either through the direct effects on the person's body or brain, or through its effects on the person's judgment, which can lead to high-risk behaviors such as violence, accidents, unprotected sex, and suicide.

As a mother, you should be alert to the warning signs of alcohol use and drug use. As noted by the American Academy of Child and Adolescent Psychiatry, look for:

- Fatigue, chronic health complaints, red/glazed eyes, and a persistent cough
- Changes in personality, mood swings, irritability, poor judgment, and low self-esteem
- Depression
- Withdrawal from the family, starting arguments, and misbehaving
- Problems in school such as multiple absences, a lack of discipline, reduced focus, and low grades
- Changes in dress, music, and friends to less conventional choices
- Trouble with the law

If you suspect a problem, contact your pediatrician, who can refer you to the appropriate health care professional.

99. What are important facts to know about sexual abuse among adolescents?

I can't tell you how many times over the years I've dealt with patients who, during their office visit, labor, or surgical procedure, have confided to me that they were sexually abused. It often comes up when a patient has a difficult time relaxing for their routine pelvic exam. They most often cite stepfathers, uncles, and male friends of the family as the perpetrators. Sometimes it was persistent abuse, and sometimes it was a one-time event.

Incidents of child sexual abuse are reported to Child Protective Services more than 80,000 times each year. This undoubtedly is a significant underestimate because many cases go unreported. Some researchers believe that 1 in 4 girls will have experienced an episode of sexual abuse before they turn 18.

Some researchers believe that 1 in 4 girls will have experienced an episode of sexual abuse before they turn 18.

Child sexual abuse is defined by the American Academy of Pediatrics as the engaging of a child in sexual activities that the child cannot comprehend, for which the child is developmentally unprepared and cannot give informed consent, and that violates the taboos of society. Sexual abuse is not limited to intercourse. Contact sexual abuse includes sexual stimulation, penetration with an object, and fondling and sexual kissing. Making of child pornography, voyeurism, sexual propositions, and exhibitionism are also forms of sexual abuse.

Although physical injury may not result, the psychological effects on a child or adolescent may be devastating. Children are not equipped to handle the intense and/or long-term emotions that sexual abuse can conjure up in them. Further, many times the adolescent knows the offender and feels an extreme sense of betrayal.

The victim also may feel conflicted about creating a problem for this person by reporting the abuse.

Sexually abused children can suffer from low self-esteem, a feeling of worthlessness, and an abnormal or distorted view of sex. They may show an unusual interest in or avoidance of all things of a sexual nature. Sleep problems, depression, delinquency, aggressive behavior, and suicide can result.

100. How can I protect my daughter against sexual abuse?

As a mother, you can help to prevent the sexual abuse of your daughter by never putting her in a position where you have even the slightest concern that an improper incident could occur; by listening carefully to, and taking seriously, any allegation she may raise about sexual abuse; and by teaching her that she should say "No" to any person who tries to inappropriately touch her and then report the incident immediately to you. Emphasize to your child that respecting adults does not mean she has to engage in blind obedience to them. Also teach your daughter to rely on her own intuition. If she becomes uncomfortable with a person or situation, she should report it to you immediately.

Build in your daughter a sense of respect for, and control over, her body. Give her the privacy she seeks when she's dressing or bathing. Don't push her to hug or kiss others if she's uncomfortable with it.

If you suspect that your daughter has been sexually abused, contact the police, Child Protective Services, or your pediatrician. Also, if appropriate, take your daughter to the local emergency room so that a specially trained professional can examine her and ensure that the necessary procedures are followed.

Child sexual abuse is a horrible crime. Don't let the perpetrator get away with it. Until he's stopped, he is likely to continue preying on girls, whether it is your daughter or someone else's.

Kama says:

An important question that parents always deliberate is "When should I allow my daughter to go out on her first date?" For my daughters, the magic age was 16, but there was a stipulation. They were required to take self-defense classes ahead of time. It gave me peace of mind to know that, should the occasion arise, she had the ability to enforce the word "No."

PART TWELVE

Conclusion

As we all know, being an adolescent girl is extraordinarily difficult in today's world. There is incredible pressure on our daughters to grow up too quickly and to become sexual beings far before their time.

Because of this, more than ever before, adolescent girls need a solid, caring, support system at home. If they don't have it, or even if they *perceive* they don't have it, they will look elsewhere for role models and for approval. Unfortunately, and sometimes even tragically, this search can lead girls far astray.

In 2003, the Girl Scout Research Institute issued a report called "Feeling Safe: What Girls Say." The researchers looked at what safety means to girls and why feeling safe matters to them. They discovered that although the majority of girls defined safety as not being *physically* hurt, almost half defined it as not having their *feelings* hurt.

Emotional safety is incredibly important to girls. Those girls who don't feel emotionally safe are far more likely to feel depressed, to have trouble making decisions, to feel less competent than their peers, to do poorly in school, and to become withdrawn and isolated.

Girls feel safest when they are with people they love and trust, such as their parents, close relatives, good friends, and dedicated teachers who have their best interests at heart. That's pretty obvious.

But it's also important to note that teens are far less likely than preteens to feel safe, both physically and emotionally. That's not only because they are more likely to face incidents of being harassed, teased, or bullied at school, but also because they worry much more than younger girls about not being able to find that special someone they can trust and talk to.

This is why your role as a mom is so vitally important. No matter what may happen in your daughter's life, *you* need to be a person she knows she can *always* trust and talk to.

As mothers, it's our sacred responsibility to provide a "safe haven"—both physically and emotionally—for our daughters. In doing so, we need to listen to them with open ears, open minds, and open hearts. Girls don't expect us to have all the answers. But they do expect us—and rightfully so—to be knowledgeable about, and sensitive to, the concerns and issues that arise during their everyday lives. Therefore, it's my hope that at least in some small way, this book has helped to enhance your knowledge of some of the important issues confronting girls today.

Empowering your daughter with the right knowledge and guidance will eventually enable her to make the right choices—even when you're nowhere around. And as your daughter ventures forth into this world full of challenges, that is one of the greatest gifts you will ever be able to give her.

Organizations

American Academy of Child and Adolescent Psychiatry

http://www.aacap.org/cs/root/facts_for_families/the_anxious_child
http://www.aacap.org/cs/root/facts_for_families/the_depressed_child

The American Academy of Pediatrics

National Headquarters
141 Northwest Point Boulevard
Elk Grove Village, IL 60007-1098
(847) 434-4000
(847) 434-8000 (Fax)
http://www.aap.org/
http://www.aap.org/advocacy/childhealthmonth/prevteensuicide.htm

American Academy of Pediatrics, Adolescent Health

http://www.aap.org/sections/adolescenthealth/default.cfm

American Cancer Society

P.O. Box 22718
Oklahoma City, OK 73123-1718
1-800-ACS-2345 (1-866-228-4327 TTY)
www.cancer.org

American College of Obstetricians and Gynecologists

P.O. Box 96920
Washington, D.C., 20090-6920
(202) 638-5577
www.acog.org
ACOG Adolescent Health Care Home Page http://www.acog.org/
    departments/dept_web.cfm?recno=7

APA Task Force Report on the Sexualization of Girls

http://www.apa.org/pi/women/programs/girls/report-full.pdf

Association of Professional Piercers (APP)

P.O. Box 1287
Lawrence, KS 66044
1-888-888-1277
http://www.safepiercing.org/

Alliance of Professional Tattooists (APT)

215 West 18th Street, Suite 210
Kansas City, MO 64108
(816) 979-1300 (Office)
(816) 979-1310 (Fax)
http://www.safe-tattoos.com/

CDC

Centers for Disease Control and Prevention
1600 Clifton Road
Atlanta, GA 30333
1-800-CDC-INFO (1-800-232-4636) TTY: 1-888-232-6348
www.cdc.gov/
Youth Risk Behavior Surveillance—United States 2007
http://www.cdc.gov/mmwr/preview/mmwrhtml/ss5704a1.htm
HPV Vaccine
http://www.cdc.gov/vaccines/vpd-vac/hpv/default.htm

Center for Young Women's Health

http://www.youngwomenshealth.org/clinicians.html
(617) 355-2994

FDA

U.S. Food and Drug Administration
10903 New Hampshire Avenue
Silver Spring, MD 20993
1-888-INFO-FDA (1-888-463-6332)
www.fda.gov/fdac/features/2000/200_tss.html

Girl Scouts of the USA

420 Fifth Avenue
New York, NY 10018-2798
1-800-478-7248
(212) 852-8000
http://www.girlscouts.org/
http://www.girlscouts.org/research/what_girls_say/personal_concerns.asp
http://www.girlscouts.org/research/publications/reviews/weighing_in.asp

Journal of Adolescent Health

http://www.journals.elsevierhealth.com/periodicals/jah

National Association of Anorexia Nervosa and Associated Eating Disorders

P.O. Box 640
Naperville, IL 60566
Help line: (630) 577-1330
Business line: (630) 577-1333
www.anad.org

North American Society for Pediatric and Adolescent Gynecology

409 12th Street, SW
Washington, D.C. 20024
(202) 863-1648
(202) 554-0453 (Fax)
http://www.naspag.org/

Society for Adolescent Medicine

1916 NW Copper Oaks Circle
Blue Springs, MO 64015
(816) 224-8010
http://www.adolescenthealth.org//AM/Template.cfm?Section=Home

Vaccine Adverse Event Reporting System (VAERS)

P.O. Box 1100
Rockville, MD 20849-1100
1-800-822-7967
1-877-721-0366 (Fax)
http://vaers.hhs.gov/index

Vaccine Safety Datalink Project
http://www.cdc.gov/vaccinesafety/Activities/VSD.html

Books

Adolescent Sexual Health Education: An Activity Source Book
Josefina J. Card and Tabitha Bennes, February 2008

Mother Daughter Wisdom: Creating a Legacy of Physical and Emotional Health
Christianne Northrup, January 2005 (Audiotape)

The Everything Parent's Guide to Raising Girls
Erika V. Shearin Karres and Rebecca Rutledge, April 2007

The Girls Report: What We Know & Need to Know about Growing Up Female
Lynn Phillips, June 1998

The Secret Lives of Teen Girls
Evelyn Resh, September 2009

Talking to Tweens
Elizabeth Hartley-Brewer, March 2005

The Teen Health Book: A Parents' Guide to Adolescent Health and Well-being
Ralph I. Lopez, April 2003

*True You! "Sometimes I Feel Ugly" and Other Truths about Growing Up:
  A Mother & Daughter Activity Book*
Randell M. Bynum, MSW, and Tonya Leslie, MA, 2006
The Girl Scout/Dove Self-Esteem Program
http://www.campaignforrealbeauty.com/dsef/download/
  BWMotherDaughterPack.pdf

When Things Get Crazy With Your Teen
Michael Bradley, September 2008

Glossary

Abstinence: The act of not participating in sexual activity.

Acetaminophen: A common over-the-counter medication used to decrease pain and reduce fevers. This medication is helpful for headaches and menstrual cramps. A common brand name is Tylenol.

Adolescence: The period of time from the onset of puberty to maturity. The World Health Organization defines this period of time as including ages 10–19. Other organizations include the ages of 8–21.

Adrenal glands: The glands in the human body responsible for producing stress response hormones, such as cortisol and adrenaline. Some androgens, or male-like hormones, are produced in the adrenal glands as well. The adrenal glands lie next to the kidneys.

Androgens: Hormones that cause masculinizing effects such as acne, increased hair growth on the face or body, enlargement of the clitoris, and deepening of the voice. In females, androgens are produced by the adrenal glands and the ovaries.

Anemia: A medical condition characterized by a low blood count, which means that the patient does not have enough red blood cells. Anemia is sometimes seen in females who experience heavy menstrual bleeding. Symptoms often include fatigue and pale skin, and may include shortness of breath and chest pain.

Anorexia nervosa: An eating disorder where the patient has an abnormal perception of her body as being too fat. Extremely low body weight, self-starvation, and excessive exercise are commonly seen in patients with this disease. Professional psychiatric help is essential for treatment of this disorder.

Antibacterial: The ability to fight off or destroy bacteria.

Antibodies: Microscopic particles in the body that fight infection. Antibodies are manufactured by the body in response to vaccinations. For example, the HPV vaccines promote antibody production to help fight off an HPV infection.

Antiperspirants: Chemicals typically used to block secretion of sweat from sweat glands under a person's arms.

Antiprostaglandins: Medications that counteract the effects of prostaglandins. Ibuprofen and naprosyn are examples of over-the-counter antiprostaglandins.

Anus: The opening of the rectum to the outside of the body.

Basal body temperature: The early morning temperature of the human body. The basal body temperature rises after ovulation occurs and can be helpful in determining the timing of intercourse for couples trying to conceive. This temperature reading is typically taken immediately upon awakening and before getting out of bed. A basal body thermometer is different from a regular thermometer and can be purchased in drugstores.

Birth control: Various forms of medications, devices, or practices that help prevent pregnancy.

Bladder infection: A common infection in women that occurs when bacteria gain entry into the bladder.

Body art: A form of art expressed on the human body. Some examples include tattoos, piercings, scarification, branding, and pubic hair designing.

Breast buds: The early breast tissue that first appears in adolescence.

Bulimia nervosa: An eating disorder characterized by consuming large amounts of food, known as binging, and then getting rid of the food, or purging, through vomiting, laxative use, or with diuretics. Those affected are usually of normal weight. Professional psychiatric help is essential for treatment of this disorder.

Cancer: An abnormal growth of cells that impairs normal body function. Also known as malignant tumors, these growths can occur in almost any organ system.

Cervical mucus: The mucus in the cervical canal that is produced by cervical glands and provides protection against pelvic infections and pregnancy. Cervical mucus changes temporarily during ovulation to enhance the chance of pregnancy.

Cervix: The organ at the lower end of the uterus that separates the uterus from the vagina. The cervix plays an important role in holding a developing fetus inside the uterus until labor begins. In addition, the cervix is the site from which samples are obtained for Pap smear testing, and it can be the site of abnormal growths such as cancer.

Chronic pelvic pain: Persistent pelvic pain that is not alleviated by usual means. Certain disorders such as endometriosis, fibroids, cysts, and pelvic adhesions can often be the cause of chronic pelvic pain, but in many cases, no cause is found.

Colposcopy: An office procedure in which the cervix is viewed through a colposcope, or magnifying instrument. A colposcopy is the test done to further evaluate the cervix after an abnormal

Pap smear. Often small biopsies are performed during this procedure.

Condom: A thin sheath, often made of latex, which is placed over the penis to capture semen for the purpose of preventing pregnancy and the transmission of infection.

Contraceptives: A general term that encompasses methods, medications, and devices to prevent pregnancy.

Cramps: A popular term used to describe the pain and discomfort originating from the uterus during the menstrual cycle. Cramps are often described as a feeling of uncomfortable pressure in the lower abdominal or back area.

Cutting: The practice of self-mutilation that involves cutting the skin with a sharp object in an attempt to ease internal pain, stress, or conflict. Typically the sites that are cut are hidden from view under clothing.

Deodorants: Products sold over-the-counter that are used to decrease body odor arising from sweat under a person's arms. Deodorants contain substances such as alcohol that kill odor-producing skin bacteria. They may be combined with antiperspirants that decrease sweat production.

Depilatories: Products such as creams, lotions, and powders that contain chemicals that remove hair. These products are commonly used to remove pubic hair and leg hair and are available over-the-counter.

Dermatitis: An irritation of the skin that can be caused by an infection or the use of a product such as a soap, lotion, or powder. The symptoms can include itching, burning, and general discomfort.

Douches: Liquids that are inserted in the vagina for the purpose of cleansing the vagina. These commonly contain vinegar and can be bought over-the-counter or made at home. Douching is not generally recommended by the medical community.

Ectopic pregnancy: A pregnancy that occurs outside of the uterine cavity. Sites can include fallopian tubes, ovaries, the cervix, and the abdomen.

Egg: Found in the ovary, the egg is a microscopic cell that is released from the ovary at the time of ovulation. The egg contains the woman's genetic material and combines with the sperm to form the embryo.

Endometriosis: A disease that is characterized by abnormal implants of cells in the female pelvis that cause pain, adhesions, and infertility. Endometriosis can run in families and usually requires surgery to diagnose. It is often treated with the birth control pill but sometimes needs stronger medications or surgical treatment.

Estradiol: An estrogen hormone produced by the ovaries that is responsible for breast development and menstrual cycles in females.

Estrogen: Refers to a number of "female" hormones found in the human body. They are produced by the ovaries, but synthetic forms also can be manufactured for use in birth control pills and for other medical purposes.

Fallopian tubes: Two long, tubular structures that are attached to the top sides of the uterus. Fertilization of the egg takes place in the fallopian tubes. Each fallopian tube lies in close proximity to each ovary.

Fertile: The ability to get pregnant without difficulty.

Fibrocystic breast disease: A very common, benign disorder that arises before a menstrual cycle and encompasses a variety of symptoms such as breast tenderness, lumpiness, and discomfort. This disease can be caused by female hormones that can stimulate very small cysts and swelling to occur in breast tissue. Other causes can be due to increased consumption of products that contain caffeine and chocolate.

Folliculitis: Inflammation of the hair follicle. Folliculitis can be painful and is caused by skin bacteria. It is often seen in the pubic hair region and appears as small pimple-like structures. Folliculitis can occur from the use of hair removal products, shaving, or waxing.

Genital warts: Warty structures on the genital region caused by the human papillomavirus. These are considered a sexually transmitted infection. Topical medications or surgical removal are used to treat them.

Genitals: A term that refers to a person's internal and external sexual organs.

Granulomas: Localized nodules of tissue that result from infection or injury.

Growth hormones: Chemicals produced by the pituitary gland that influence metabolism and cause growth of organs.

Growth spurt: A period of rapid growth in height, weight, and muscle mass that takes place in adolescence, typically between the ages of 11–14 for girls, and 12–16 for boys.

Gynecologist: A medical doctor who specializes in the care of women and the treatment of diseases that affect their sexual organs.

Hormones: Chemicals produced by an organ that have an effect on other organs or cells in the human body.

Hypoallergenic: A product that has a low likelihood of causing an allergic reaction.

Ibuprofen: A commonly used over-the-counter antiprostaglandin medication that helps menstrual cramps. Two common brand names are Motrin and Advil.

Infertility: The inability to get pregnant without assistance.

Jaundice: A yellowing of the skin and eyes often caused by liver disease.

Keloids: A scar that extends beyond the site of the original wound and can grow over time. These scars can be hereditary and occur more often in African Americans, Latinos, and Asians. They commonly occur around piercing sites.

Labia: The folds of tissue on the vulva. There are two sets of labia, the labia majora (outer) and the labia minora (inner).

Lactobacillus bacteria: The "good" bacteria found in the vagina that are responsible for maintaining a normal vaginal environment. These bacteria help fight off bad bacteria that cause vaginal and urinary tract infections.

Lymph nodes: Small bean-like structures that contain white blood cells and help fight infection. They are scattered throughout the body.

Menarche: The initial onset of menstrual cycles.

Menstrual cycle: The monthly episode of vaginal bleeding that can last for up to a week.

Menstrual flow: The amount of blood that exits the vagina during a menstrual cycle.

Menstruate: The release of the menstrual blood from the uterus and out of the vagina.

Menstruation: The breakdown and shedding of the uterine lining resulting in the menstrual period.

Monogamous: Being in a relationship between two people with no other partners.

Naprosyn: A common over-the-counter, antiprostaglandin product that is used for menstrual cramps, headaches, and other pains. One example is Aleve.

Oral sex: A sexual act involving oral stimulation of the genital area.

Ovulation: The release of the egg from the ovary that occurs monthly. The egg is then picked up by the fallopian tube and awaits fertilization.

Pap smear: The sample of cells taken from the cervix during a speculum exam. Historically, the cells were smeared on a slide for interpretation in the lab. These days, the cells are released

into a vial with liquid, cleansed, and then interpreted.

Parabens: Chemical preservatives found in many cosmetic products and deodorants.

Pelvic abscess: A localized area of pus in the pelvic region.

Pelvic exam: An examination of the female reproductive organs. This exam can include an external inspection of the genital region, a speculum exam of the vagina and cervix, and/or a manual exam of the internal genital organs, i.e., the uterus and cervix.

Period: Refers to the periodic bleeding that occurs monthly from the uterus. Also known as the menstrual cycle.

Pituitary gland: A gland in the brain that is responsible for producing various hormones. The pituitary gland secretes hormones that stimulate thyroid function, ovulation, breast milk production, growth and metabolism, and adrenal gland function.

Placebo: A substance that contains no medicine. "Sugar pills" found in packs of birth control pills are placebo pills.

PMS: An abbreviation that refers to premenstrual syndrome. PMS refers to the period of time preceding the menstrual period where, due to elevated levels of progesterone, symptoms of bloating, moodiness, irritability, acne, and breast tenderness are more prevalent.

Polycystic ovarian syndrome: A common hormonal disorder seen in young women and female adolescents that involves a variety of symptoms. Classic symptoms include infrequent menstrual cycles, acne, excessive hair growth, obesity, and a cystic appearance of the ovaries on sonograms. This syndrome can run in families, but the exact cause is unknown. Elevated glucose, or sugar, levels can be detected. A common treatment is the birth control pill.

Precancerous: A condition in which there is the potential that a cancer will form. Precancerous cells on the cervix, if left untreated, may have the ability to form cervical cancer.

Progesterone: Progesterone is produced by the ovaries following ovulation and is responsible for preparing the lining of the uterus for pregnancy. When progesterone levels decline, menstruation occurs. Some of the side effects of progesterone include moodiness, headaches, acne, bloating, and depression. Synthetic forms of progesterone are found in hormonal methods of birth control.

Prolactin: A hormone secreted by the pituitary gland that stimulates breast milk production. Elevated levels of the prolactin hormone can be caused by growths on the pituitary gland, breast stimulation, and certain medications. An elevated prolactin hormone level can interfere with ovulation and prevent menstrual cycles from occurring.

Prostaglandins: A group of naturally occurring hormonal substances that have a widespread effect on the human body. One type of prostaglandin is produced by the uterus and causes contractions of the uterine muscle. High levels of prostaglandin have been associated with painful menstrual cramps.

Puberty: The period of time in which a child undergoes physiological and emotional changes that help her/him develop into a young adult capable of reproducing. These changes can start occurring as early as the age of eight in girls and nine in boys, and are due to elevations in hormones that cause development of sexual organs and growth spurts.

Safe sex: Sexual activity that incorporates the use of birth control and condoms to minimize the risk of pregnancy and transmission of sexually transmitted infections.

Sanitary pads: A pad of absorbent material worn to absorb menstrual blood.

Self-objectification: The American Psychological Association uses this term to describe young women who learn to think of and treat their own bodies simply as objects of others' desires.

Semen: The fluid containing sperm that is released from the penis during ejaculation. This fluid helps the sperm reach the egg for fertilization.

Sexual intercourse: The insertion of the erect male penis into the female vagina.

Sexualization: The American Psychological Association defines this term as including one or more of the following criteria: a person's value is determined solely by his or her sexual appeal or behavior; a person is held to a standard whereby only physically attractive people are deemed to be worthy sexual beings; a person is viewed only as a "thing" for another's sexual use; and/or sexuality is inappropriately imposed upon a person.

Sexually transmitted disease (STD): Also known as sexually transmitted infection (STI), or venereal disease (VD), this category includes any infection that can be transmitted from one person to another through any sexual contact, including oral sex.

Sperm: The cells in the semen that fertilize the female egg. Sperm contain the father's genetic material.

Spotting: A very light, scanty amount of bleeding from the vagina that can be bright red or dark brown in color. Often this kind of bleeding is seen at the very beginning or the very end of a woman's menstrual cycle.

Staph bacteria: A common type of bacteria normally found on skin surfaces that can cause infections. The *staphylococcus aureus* bacteria can produce a toxin that is the cause of Toxic Shock Syndrome.

Tampon: A plug of absorbent material placed in the vagina to prevent menstrual blood from coming out.

Thelarche: The development of breast tissue in an adolescent.

Toxic Shock Syndrome (TSS): A rare and potentially lethal illness caused by toxins excreted from bacteria. Historically linked to tampon use, Toxic Shock Syndrome can occur anytime these toxins have an opportunity to gain access into the human body. Symptoms include fever, a drop in blood pressure, rash, peeling of skin from palms and soles, nausea and vomiting, liver inflammation, renal failure, low blood platelets, and confusion.

Toxin: A poisonous product of animal and plant cells or bacteria that causes tissue damage and antibody formation.

Tweens: Refers to adolescents who are no longer considered "children," but who are not yet teenagers.

Urethra: The short tube that opens just in front of the vagina. It carries urine from the bladder to the outside.

Uterus: A hollow, pear-shaped organ in the pelvis where a developing fetus grows. The lower part is attached to the cervix. The lining of the uterus sheds monthly as the menstrual period.

Vagina: The muscular, tube-like organ that extends from the uterus and cervix to the outside of the body. The opening is located in between the urethra and the anus. It is lined with glands that produce mucous secretions.

Vaginal discharge: A mucus-like substance coming from the vagina. A small amount of non-odorous discharge can be normal. A large amount of discharge accompanied by itching, odor, or unusual color can indicate an infection.

Vulva: The external female genital organs that include the labia majora, labia minora, clitoris, Bartholins glands, and the opening to the vagina (vestibule).

Yeast infection: One of the most common vaginal infections among women. This infection is not sexually transmitted. Yeast is commonly present in the vagina in very small amounts. A change in the balance of the vaginal flora often caused by taking an antibiotic will cause the yeast to overgrow and symptoms of itching and discharge can occur.

Index

Index

Index